Speaking of Dying

of related interest

Passionate Supervision
Edited by Robin Shohet
ISBN 978 1 84310 556 5

The Art of Helping Others
Being Around, Being There, Being Wise
Heather Smith and Mark Smith
ISBN 978 1 84310 638 8

A Bolt from the Blue
Coping with Disasters and Acute Traumas
Salli Saari
Translated by Annira Silver
ISBN 978 1 84310 313 4

Grandad's Ashes
Walter Smith
ISBN 978 1 84310 517 6

The Creative Arts in Palliative Care
Edited by Nigel Hartley and Malcolm Payne
ISBN 978 1 84310 591 6

Prayer in Counselling and Psychotherapy
Exploring a Hidden Meaningful Dimension
Peter Madsen Gubi
Foreword by Brian Thorne
ISBN 978 1 84310 519 0

Supporting the Child and the Family in Paediatric Palliative Care
Erica Brown
With Brian Warr
Foreword by Dr. Sheila Shribman, National Clinical Director for Children, Maternity Services, Department of Health
ISBN 978 1 84310 181 9

Dying, Bereavement and the Healing Arts
Edited by Gillie Bolton
Foreword by Baroness Professor Ilora Finlay of Llandaff
ISBN 978 1 84310 516 9

Speaking of Dying

A Practical Guide to Using
Counselling Skills in Palliative Care

Louis Heyse-Moore

Foreword by Colin Murray Parkes

Jessica Kingsley Publishers
London and Philadelphia

The author and publishers are grateful to the proprietors listed below for permission to quote the following material:

From CANCER vol 53, no 10 (suppl), 1984. Copyright © 1984 American Cancer Society. This material is reproduced with permission of Wiley-Liss, Inc., a subsidiary of John Wiley & Sons, Inc. From *How to Win Friends and Influence People* by Dale Carnegie, published by Vermilion. Reprinted by permission of the Random House Group Ltd. From *Kitchen Table Wisdom* by Rachel Naomi Remen, published by Pan Macmillan, London. Copyright © Remen 1997. From *The Words to Say It* by Marie Cardinal. Reprinted by permission of The Women's Press Ltd. Figure 5.1 from *The Act of Will* by R. Assagioli. Brantford, ON: Turnstone Press. Reprinted by permission. Table 6.1 reprinted by permission of The Samaritans and the British Medical Journal.

First published in 2009
by Jessica Kingsley Publishers
116 Pentonville Road
London N1 9JB, UK
and
400 Market Street, Suite 400
Philadelphia, PA 19106, USA

www.jkp.com

Library of Congress Cataloging in Publication Data
Heyse-Moore, Louis.
      Speaking of dying : a practical guide to using counselling skills in palliative care / Louis Heyse-Moore ; foreword by Colin Murray Parkes.
        p. ; cm.
      Includes bibliographical references.
      ISBN 978-1-84310-678-4 (pb : alk. paper) 1. Palliative treatment--Psychological aspects. 2. Terminal care--Psychological aspects. 3. Counseling. I. Title. II. Title: Practical guide to using counselling skills in palliative care.
      [DNLM: 1. Palliative Care--psychology. 2. Attitude to Death. 3. Counseling--methods. 4. Terminal Care--psychology. WB 310 H621s 2009]
      R726.8.H49 2009
      616'.029--dc22
                          2008014725

British Library Cataloguing in Publication Data
A CIP catalogue record for this book is available from the British Library

ISBN 978 1 84310 678 4

Contents

Be what you is, cuz if you be what you ain't, then you ain't what you is.

Epitaph on a tombstone in Boothill Cemetery in Tombstone, Arizona

(Campbell 1990, p.xxiv)

To Joan

And to Matthew, Dominique and Gabrielle

Acknowledgements

I would like to thank the following for their advice: Pam Firth on family issues, Rev. Geoffrey Brown on spiritual matters, Dominique Heyse-Moore on race, and Jacqui Feld for our many conversations on staff support; also the training team and my training group at Re.Vision for all I have learnt from them about the counselling relationship.

I would also like to express a debt of gratitude to all the patients and clients I have worked with, some of whose stories appear in this book. They have taught me more than any book could do.

Foreword

Human beings are the only creatures who know that we will die. All species have evolved with powerful mental and physical equipment that enables us to survive, at least until we have reached reproductive age and handed on our genes. Our brains evolved to avoid death not to face it. We are not programmed for death, but for life.

From the moment of our conception we are all dying. Yet there are no schools for dying. Faced with the biggest threat in our lives we say nothing or we lie. 'Die my dear doctor? That's the last thing I shall do'.[1] It follows that it is difficult to speak of dying.

But Dr Heyse-Moore invites us to do just that. He has taken the well-tried lessons of counselling and developed them for all those who set out to help people who are approaching the end of their lives. He is well-qualified to do this because he draws on long experience as a Palliative Care Physician and caring doctor. As one who worked alongside him at St Joseph's Hospice for many years I can testify to the validity of the examples he gives; they are taken from life, not psychological theories.

Speaking of Dying is not as brutal as the title suggests. Dr Heyse-Moore knows full well the harm that we can do by battering defences against the facts of death that have been cultivated over many years. That's why members of the caring professions need all the counselling skills that we can muster. Readers of this book will end up feeling less helpless in the face of death but we should not expect to find communication easy. 'What can we say?' Once we think we know what to say we are wrong. Rather this book will help us to learn when to speak of dying and when not to, what not to say and when to keep silent and wait patiently for what gliding instructors call an 'up-draught'. We must start from wherever the other person may be and we must take the time and trouble to discover the language with which this person speaks about death and dying, the

---

1   Allegedly the last words of Lord Palmerstone.

assumptions they make, and their needs and wishes to speak or not to speak.

Cancers and other life-threatening illnesses invade families as well as patients. We are all threatened by the death of those we love. Consequently the family is an important part of the unit of care both before and, often, after the patient has died. Even in this book, which is directed primarily at the care of the patient, the family cannot and is not left out of the equation. Support for the family is support for the patient and *vice versa*.

'Doctor, Doctor, shall I die? Yes, my child and so shall I.' We are all dying and the person in the bed is only one step closer than you or I. The care of patients and families threatened with death can be hard for the carers as well as the cared-for. Who cares for the counsellors? Louis Heyse-Moore leaves this question to the end of the book where it belongs, not only because our patients come first, but also because, by the time we are expected to turn the spotlight on ourselves, we know what to expect to find.

The care of people at times of death can be the most painful, but also the most rewarding aspect of medical care. If we can acknowledge our own pain and support each other when necessary, we shall find that, however sad and sometimes tragic our work may be, on balance the successes outweigh the failures. Not everybody dies happy in a hospice, hospital or home, even with the best of care, but our attempts to speak of dying, with our patients, with their families and with each other, usually make things better rather than worse, and sometimes turn disaster into triumph.

Dr Colin Murray Parkes
Life President of Cruse Bereavement Care

Introduction

It was 1973. I had just qualified and was working as a house surgeon. I hadn't had any training in communication skills – apart from being told to behave professionally. All the doctors I worked with dissembled or lied if asked about the diagnosis by a cancer patient, so I did the same, though I didn't feel comfortable about it. One day, a woman was admitted with a newly diagnosed cancer. She had previously had, unusually, two other primary cancers. As I clerked her in, I remember thinking I didn't want to dodge questions about diagnosis any more. It was still a shock, though, when she asked me if it was cancer. My heart rate shot up, but I couldn't find it in me to avoid her question. 'Yes,' was all I said. She began to cry and asked, after a while, why it kept coming back. Of course I had no answer, but I remember feeling a deep compassion for her plight and also a sense that we had met, person to person. She wanted to have that information about her cancer and it felt right to respect her wish, even though I was stepping outside usual medical practice. I wish I had had more skills to support her psychologically as she came to terms with her illness (Heyse-Moore 2007).

I hope this story says something about why I'm writing a book on counselling skills in palliative care. First, from my own experience working for many years in palliative medicine alongside colleagues from different clinical disciplines, it is clear to me that these skills are essential to providing good care for the dying. Second, I wish when I was starting in this field, there had been a guide to talking to the terminally ill written by someone familiar with the many problems they present. This book is an attempt to meet that need.

There is, of course, a spectrum of attitudes in different clinical disciplines to using counselling skills. For social workers, they are a basic part of their approach to working with the dying. At the other end of the scale, doctors have traditionally received little or no training in this area. It is true that teaching on communication skills is now part of the medical school curricula in the United Kingdom, a radical change from when I was a student. However, when I have talked with junior doctors whom I have supervised clinically, it became clear that, while they were taught the essentials of good communication, they were taught no more than this. Though this served well enough for the majority of patients, it was insufficient for difficult clinical situations – patients in crisis, acute psychoses, major depression and so on. Junior doctors may still be faced with the initial management of such cases, often unaided. Furthermore, if one of the medical team is interested in talking with patients with advanced cancer about their illness, other doctors, including some consultants, finding this area difficult, may devolve this responsibility to him.

This book is intended to be useful to practitioners in all disciplines working clinically in palliative care, whether as part of that specialty or in general clinical settings that involve care of those with advanced or incurable illnesses. Which disciplines am I talking about? I'll mention doctors first – my original profession. I know from first-hand experience the difficulties junior doctors face in being left to deal with the terminally ill without support. I had to build up my own skills in this area slowly and painfully, and with many mistakes. I hope this book will help doctors travelling this road. It is also addressed to nurses, chaplains, physiotherapists, complementary therapists and occupational therapists. Volunteers, particularly those who provide bereavement support, but also others who come into contact with patients, may find it useful. Social workers will often have had their own psychological training, but even so, they and counsellors should find the slant on the special issues pertaining to palliative care will still be of interest to them. I am not a nurse or social worker or minister, so my insights as to their approaches to using counselling skills are guided by the many people I have worked with in these fields.

Dame Cicely Saunders, the founder of St Christopher's Hospice, taught the concept of *Total Pain*, made up of physical, mental, social and

[handwritten top: HEALTH-CARE-WORKER ⟶ A Clinician > Kline "Bed"]
[handwritten: ↳ Ministers their expertise near/on patient's Bed! — w/ Family present! — (A)]

Table I.1 Total suffering

[handwritten: OR TOTAL PAIN / Multi-MODAL Approach?]

BODY *[handwritten: → Physical Symptoms, Pain, Physical Sensation, Bodily changes, Tumours, loss of Body parts, loss of Function (Stroke) Heart Attack.]*   Including not only physical symptoms such as pain, but also any body sensation, bodily changes such as skin tumours, loss of a body part such as mastectomy and loss of function such as a stroke.
PSYCHE/MIND *[handwritten: ⇒ Mental suff, Emot. distress,]*   All aspects of mental suffering such as emotional distress, loss, stress, nightmares and psychopathologies. *[handwritten: Imagined threats of: etc.]*
RELATIONSHIPS/SOCIAL   Including conflict, estrangement and loss related to family, friends, colleagues and work.
SPIRIT *[handwritten: → loss of: Mean, Purpos, Sign. (Belief), Isolation/Inner Darkness]*   For example loss of purpose, meaning or belief; inner darkness, isolation.

[handwritten right margin: /BAD PERSON Hell ← Punished ✓ No Hope.]

[handwritten: Clinician → Gk "Kline" → BED ⟹ Patient's Bed — Family Present]

spiritual elements. This is a key idea in understanding how pain is not just physical but affected by these other modalities too. Repeatedly, for example, I have seen how formerly resistant physical pain improved when a concomitant depression was also addressed. I'd like to suggest a broad understanding of this theme, as shown in Table I.1. These different aspects of suffering in the dying will be elaborated further in Part 2 of this book.

Our response to total suffering, to be effective, needs to be addressed to the whole person, an holistic approach, to employ a widely and loosely used, but nevertheless apt, phrase. Just as suffering is multimodal, so must our therapeutic stance be, and this may include the input of many different clinical disciplines. It is of little use addressing an individual's emotional distress if she has uncontrolled, severe, physical pain which occupies all her attention. Similarly, it is insufficient to treat a person's physical pain and ignore her emotional suffering. Counselling skills are pertinent to every facet of holistic care, whether physical, psychological, relational or spiritual.

To me, the generic expression 'health care worker' is unwieldy, so I've chosen instead to use the term 'clinician' when referring collectively to all clinical disciplines. It comes from the Greek, *kline*, meaning 'bed', and reflects the fact that so many interactions with the dying patient and her family take place around the bed.

Much clinical writing emphasises the rational approach of science. This is obviously foundational and yet it doesn't capture the essence of an actual encounter using counselling skills. Advice to be empathetic or to listen prompts the question: how? I'll therefore also make use of an approach that addresses the qualitative through stories, imagery and the feelings. It is popular now to see the left cerebral hemisphere of the brain as the mediator of logic and the right as creative, visual and comprehending wholes. While this is an oversimplification of the complexities of our psychological processes, since both hemispheres are involved in both sets of activities, combining these approaches can only enhance the richness of the material here presented. Experience is the best teacher so I'll use clinical examples and literary excerpts which illustrate a particular point. References to patients or relatives have been made anonymous by changing identifying details.

What is the essence of the counselling process? Albert Schweitzer once made this statement: 'Each patient carries his own doctor inside him. They come to us not knowing that truth. We are at our best when we give the doctor who resides within each patient a chance to go to work' (Cousins 1979, p.69).

While he was speaking ostensibly from a medical perspective, something similar applies in psychological therapy – it is about assisting the individual to discover his own inner healing, an avenue still open to him even when he is dying.

The initial theme of the book will be about reviewing counselling skills and this will be followed by a section on common issues in palliative care where counselling skills are needed, such as breaking bad news and euthanasia. It is intended more as a practical handbook than an academic study, but references are given for further reading.

I will use the term 'patient' when writing from the point of view of a clinician, and 'client' when referring to formal counselling. When gender isn't already specified I will alternate between masculine and feminine pronouns.

ALTHEA – A FICTIONAL CASE-HISTORY

To illustrate the use of counselling skills, I will also include a fictional case-history, including transcripts, of conversations with a patient whom I will call Althea. She is 35 years old and has breast cancer with bone

[handwritten margin notes: "CADUCEUS → Held By ASKLEPIOS", "SNAKE", "The moving of the cancer to another part!"]

metastases. She teaches languages at a secondary school. She is married to Winston who is mixed race and a lawyer; they have two young children, Rachel, aged eight, and Jack, aged six. The character of Althea reflects many different patients I have talked to with advanced cancer.

ROOTS OF HEALTHCARE PRACTICE:

[handwritten note: "A) AsKlePious → Mystery Tradition Approach to Illness, B) Hippocrates → Naturalistic Approach to illness,"]

If we go back to health care in Ancient Greece (Achteberg 2002), which was the forerunner of our modern clinical practice and the different clinical disciplines involved, we find two strands. The older is that of Asklepios, who probably existed historically and was later deified. He represented the mystery tradition and many temples were founded in his name, which could be regarded as the first holistic therapy centres. The temple at Epidaurus, for example, had a theatre for staging plays to induce *katharsis*, the release of emotions. These 'Asklepia' focused on the use of dreams for both diagnosis and treatment. The maidens who helped the ill person prepare for the sleep ritual in the temples were called *therapae*, a possible etymological source for the modern term 'therapist'. Asklepios was portrayed as holding a rustic staff with a serpent entwined on it (serpents were considered sacred and kept in the temples). This image, the *caduceus*, is still used as a symbol of the medical profession, even though some of its present-day members might find themselves out of step with the Asklepian approach.

The other strand is represented by Hippocrates. While he was trained in and practised the Asklepian tradition, he also focused on a naturalistic approach to illness. His was a common-sense, down-to-earth methodology, and is the ancestor of the way much of medicine is practised now. His Hippocratic Oath contained such wisdom it is still well known today, even if doctors no longer swear the oath.

It is clear that the Asklepian tradition has all but disappeared in many branches of medicine, though it does find some place in psychiatry, and, more recently, in palliative care. Other clinical disciplines such as nursing and social work are more in sympathy with this paradigm. It is now primarily the province of psychological therapists who are usually non-clinical, although they may at times also be social workers, nurses or doctors.

While the two strands worked well together in Ancient Greece, the situation is not so harmonious today. The validity of the qualitative approach of many psychological therapies has been questioned, particularly in medical circles. This scepticism perhaps relates to the almost exclusive focus of present-day medicine on a logical, scientific, quantitative methodology. Clearly this has achieved remarkable results, but it does mean that the qualitative approach which speaks to the individuality, the uniqueness of each person, has taken a back seat.

So, when we use counselling skills in palliative care, we are bringing in something of the other, overlooked strand of our healing tradition, providing a more inclusive approach to our patients, perceiving them not just as machines to be engineered, but also as people with thoughts, feelings, hopes, dreams and relationships. D.H. Lawrence who died of tuberculosis, which was as dreaded in his time as cancer is now, wrote several poems of his last illness. He had this to say in his poem 'Healing' (1994, p.513):

I am not a mechanism, an assembly of various sections.
And it is not because the mechanism is working wrongly, that I am ill.
I am ill because of wounds to the soul, to the deep emotional self –
and the wounds to the soul take a long, long time, only time can help
and patience, and a certain difficult repentance,
long difficult repentance, realisation of life's mistake, and the freeing
oneself *Repeating the beat up! → makes one sick*
from the endless repetition of the mistake *that is why*
which mankind at large has chosen to sanctify. *illness occurs & prevails!*

Part 1
Fundamentals
of Counselling Skills

[handwritten top margin:] PALLIATION → To cloak, To cover.
→ Palliative Medicine Focuses on: A) Symptom Control
B) Pain Management
C) Make Pain-Free Experience Create

[right side handwritten:] D) Provide A Better Quality of Life In Ay Patients EoL Experience.

Terminology

[handwritten:] → Over: Pain ⎫ Terminal (w/ Pain meds!
Disease ⎬ — Morph. ✓
Illness ⎭ — Doma.
— Vicodyn
— Percocept
— etc

PALLIATION *[handwritten:]* → To cloak, cover, shield, envelope

This term comes from the Latin *palliare* meaning 'to cloak'. It is used where clinical treatment is provided to reduce the impact of an illness, not to cure it – thus morphine is prescribed to reduce the pain of an incurable cancer, *[handwritten:]* or Any disease!

Palliative care is the term applied to all clinical care for patients whose illness is advanced, advancing, incurable, life-threatening and, *[handwritten:]* Terminal symptomatic. There is, too, a move now to include patients earlier on in the course of a long-term illness. At present, over 90 per cent of patients admitted to palliative care units have cancer. However, non-malignant illnesses, such as end-stage kidney, heart or lung failure, or motor neurone disease, for example, are also suitable *[handwritten:]* for Palliative Care Treatment!

[left margin handwritten:] Covering ε Cloakling Pain. ε Symptoms is Key Here!

Palliative medicine is the medical specialty which provides care for these patients. It focuses on: symptom control but also addresses psychological, social and spiritual distress in conjunction with other clinical disciplines. This team work is essential to success in managing these issues.

THE PSYCHE

There are many different models which map the psyche, the seat of all our mental faculties (Assagioli 1975, p.17; Jung 1964, p.171; Rycroft 1995). Perhaps the best known is Freud's triadic view of the instinctual id, the conscious ego and the supervisory *[handwritten:]* unconscious super-ego. For our purposes the most important practical distinction is between the conscious and unconscious. Consciousness is what we are aware of at any moment. The unconscious is all the rest and is vast. Some of it is easily accessible – for example a conversation with a friend yesterday – and some not – such as memories of childhood abuse. Jung (1969, p.141) had this to say:

> It [the psyche] reaches so far beyond the boundaries of consciousness that the latter could be compared to an island in the ocean. Whereas the island is small and narrow, the ocean is immensely wide and deep and contains a life infinitely surpassing, in kind and degree, anything known on the island.

Once, I flew at night from Los Angeles to Hawaii. For five hours the plane traversed the vast, moonlit Pacific Ocean and it seemed a miracle to me that it was able to find our destination, a tiny dot in the immensity of the sea. I understood then something of what Jung meant. We like to think we are rational beings; the truth is not so simple. The unconscious influences us in myriad ways – through dreams, fantasies, unexpected feelings and Freudian slips for example. One woman with advanced lung cancer told me she would be fine if she could just stop having panic attacks. She wasn't prepared to let in awareness of a connection between her fear and her diagnosis, underlying which was the deeper fear of death. In this context, Jung described the Shadow (Storr 1998, pp.414–23), by which he meant everything that we refuse to acknowledge about ourselves and so repress into the unconsciousness. As indicated above, death is often a shadow figure and is typically represented as a terrifying, skeletal presence, cloaked in black and wielding a scythe. An alternative image of death as a kindly angel is less familiar - except, perhaps, in graveyards.

The Shadow does not go away, however, if repressed; it returns later, often in disguised form. Thus, bereaved people who suppress their grief and try quickly to return to normal may find they develop psychological symptoms such as anxiety or insomnia months or even years later.

COUNSELLING

This has been variously defined. Essential elements include the following:

- It is a professional activity that is based on and works through the interpersonal relationship between counsellor and client.

- The client brings an issue, looking for resolution. While this may be apparently external ('My partner won't talk to me') it is ultimately about the client's internal attitude to the problem. Not surprisingly, the presenting issue is likely to hide a different and deeper difficulty. For example, insomnia may be due to recurrent nightmares because of childhood parental violence.

- The client is at the centre. It is he who works out a deeper understanding of himself. It is he who decides what changes, if any, to make in his life. The counsellor is there to facilitate this process.

THERAPY AND THE MEDICAL MODEL

The medical model views the patient as being ill, having some physical pathology, such as cancer or heart disease. It sees its task as both diagnostic – to discover what is wrong – and curative – as far as possible to put it right. It has been applied both to physical illnesses, where it often works well, and to psychological conditions, where there is, at times, controversy as to its appropriateness.

While some forms of therapy, such as cognitive behavioural therapy, subscribe to this model, many do not. Where the medical model would see a symptom such as depression or panic attacks as an illness to be got rid of, many psychologies would see them as warning signs that the individual's life is out of balance. As such, they can be also be viewed as useful, though distressing, messengers which need to be listened to and their meaning understood. An example, which is not uncommon, would be of a woman who goes to see her GP with depression. The quick answer would be to prescribe antidepressants. Further enquiry, however, may reveal that her much loved husband died two years ago and she suppressed this grief by plunging back into her work to try to forget her pain. Her depression is telling her that she needs to grieve in order to heal. Both approaches have something to offer and – significantly – may be synergistic in combination.

COUNSELLING SKILLS

The skills that counsellors use can be employed in a wide variety of settings by other professionals such as doctors, nurses, teachers or managers, or in supporting a friend or colleague. There are, though, differences between this informal approach and formal counselling (Culley and Bond 2004, p.6; Heyse-Moore 2007).

Role

Counselling is a professional activity. However, when counselling skills are used by clinicians, they have to combine this with their other roles. For doctors, this will be diagnostics and treatment; for nurses, assessing nursing needs such as dependency. It took practice for me to know when to change from the closed-ended questions of a medical history to the open-ended ones used in counselling. It helps to take your cue from the patient. Monitoring his emotional state is part of this. Both intense, and deadened, feelings reveal an emotionally charged complex which is either being expressed or suppressed. The doctor may also need to prescribe, and the nurse administer, treatments with side-effects, such as chemotherapy, and at the same time support the patient through his fears about this very treatment.

One way clinicians avoid talking to patients about feelings is by keeping along the track of asking closed questions. Thus, if the patient comments: 'I'm feeling frightened', avoidant responses might be: 'Are you taking your tranquillisers?' or: 'I'll get the chaplain to talk to you'.

Authority

The counsellor has no formal authority over the client. In a sense this is true of clinicians; however, patients do invest clinicians, and doctors in particular, with authority and expect to receive advice which they will often accept. Doctors willingly take on this role and tend to expect compliance. Some patients, especially the elderly, are so used to this, they have difficulty in deciding when presented with a range of treatment options. 'What would you do, doctor?' they say to me, struggling with taking responsibility for their illness and its management. It takes time to work through with them what they feel about the various treatments but it is time well spent which they appreciate - they are being treated as responsible adults after all. A few have a deep fear of making choices and enlist a family member to decide for them. It is, it must be remembered, a temptation for busy doctors, say on emergency take, to save time by informing the patient what her treatment will be and moving on quickly before questions are voiced. We would, however, not expect other professionals such as lawyers to behave in this way. Doctors are no exception.

[handwritten margin notes: Timing / # of sessions / payment / confidentiality / goals]

Contracts

Counsellors set up an explicit agreement with their clients, often written. This will include timings, number of sessions, payment, confidentiality and goals. Of these, perhaps the last is most likely to be explored in a clinical interview using counselling skills. Confidentiality is usually implicit, though patients are often asked nowadays if they give permission for their clinical details to be discussed with family or close friends. Palliative care units normally work on a team confidentiality basis, that clinical information is shared between members of the clinical team on a 'need to know' basis. One way of telling patients about this is to provide an information leaflet when they are admitted.

Timings

Counsellors agree this clearly with their client: 'We will meet once a week for an hour on Wednesdays at 2 pm for a total of eight sessions. We will review our work during the last session'. Out-patient appointments are, perhaps, the closest equivalent in clinical work. Because of smaller patient numbers, palliative care avoids the chronic problems found in hospitals of delayed, rushed appointments and seeing a different doctor at each visit. On the ward, patients take a passive role, waiting for the doctor to do her rounds, or for the nurse or social worker to see them when their professional schedule allows. Meetings may last anywhere between five minutes and two hours or more, though discussions involving support often last considerably less than the counselling hour because of patient frailty.

In palliative care, then, the hour-a-week counselling model isn't usually appropriate. Many patients are within days or weeks of death; they can't wait a week for the next session. Indeed they may require intensive, even daily, input. One patient with a brain tumour talked about coming to terms with his illness for five hours one day with three different members of staff – a multicentric, multidisciplinary use of counselling skills.

Professional support

Counsellors are obliged to have regular professional supervision to maintain their clinical and ethical standards. The same applies for social workers in palliative care. Doctors in palliative medicine do receive informal supervision on ward rounds, but formal supervision is often not available. My experience has been that junior doctors readily accept this and find it helpful, provided the facilitator has the appropriate skills, which includes both clinical management and psychological support. Similarly, nurses may or may not receive clinical supervision, although their regular daily handovers may have a supportive element to them.

Process

Counselling is based on the relationship that develops between the counsellor and client. Building on the trust this engenders, the client gradually deepens her self-understanding – how it is that she feels, thinks and acts the way she does. She may decide, supported by her counsellor, to make changes in her life, a mysterious process that may take moments or years.

In palliative care, as indicated above, the slow pace of counselling is often not feasible. Furthermore, the patients have not agreed to formal counselling; in fact they may know little of it and distrust the process. So the support provided is a mixed bag – counselling skills, advice, coaching, symptom control and provision of resources – with an emphasis on short-term goals. It can be useful that it is the doctor or nurse providing the help – this is a socially sanctioned way of getting support without the stigma of being mentally ill.

Usually, meetings involving the doctor include other clinical disciplines, often nurses. Family may be present. At the next meeting, there may be a different configuration of people involved. For this reason, clear notes and handovers, especially between the doctors, nurses and social workers are essential to ensure the whole team keeps track of what has been said in meetings with the patient and his family, and where they are in their inner processes – be it about the illness or their relationships.

Some patients are in crisis with a breakdown of their psychological defences and so may be much more open to counselling support and to change.

The focus

In counselling, the client is at the centre. The context of her presenting issues provides a perspective about herself for her and the counsellor to work with. The needs of others are considered insofar as they relate to the client.

The clinician using counselling skills has a dual perspective: both the client and his context – for example, his symptoms, his psychological distress, possible conflicts with his family or complaints about care provision. The clinician can't be solely the patient's advocate to the exclusion of all else but will need to balance this with the other factors involved. Thus, I remember a husband who was bed-bound and determined to go home without extra nursing support. He would not take account of the fact that his wife was frail and elderly and not able to provide the nursing care he needed. She felt frightened that he would be sent home and guilty that she could not give him what he wanted. The work here was with both him and his wife towards an acceptance of the unpalatable but unavoidable facts.

PSYCHOTHERAPY / OR Just → Counselling

There is no generally accepted distinction between counselling and psychotherapy.

- Some people use these terms interchangeably. Both modalities may involve work at considerable depth.

- There may be specific trainings in psychotherapy, such as gestalt or psychodynamic therapies.

- Counselling is more likely to focus on particular issues or adjustment to life events such as bereavement, whereas psychotherapy is more likely to be concerned with a deeper remodelling of the individual's personality and her relationship to her core Self. Both approaches may work with the unconscious, but this will tend to be more intensive in psychotherapy.

- Psychotherapists are more likely to work at greater depth, using specialised skills, with very disturbed individuals and see them more often over a longer time scale.

PSYCHOANALYSIS

This is the therapy beloved of cartoonists in which the client lies on a couch and the analyst sits anonymously behind him. It refers to the treatment and psychological origins of neuroses as formulated by Freud and his followers (Rycroft 1995, p.143). It is also used informally to describe Jungian and Adlerian therapy. Like psychotherapy, it is an in-depth process in which the client may see the analyst several times a week for many years. This implies considerable expense. Such an approach is obviously unsuitable for the dying but might be appropriate for someone early in his cancer journey who wishes to explore himself in depth and who has enough money to do so. However, psychoanalytic concepts (Goldie and Desmarais 2005) have been used successfully to provide psychotherapy for cancer patients in an oncology hospital, whether for one meeting or regular sessions.

PROJECTION

This is 'the process whereby an unconscious quality or characteristic of one's own is perceived and reacted to in an outer object or person' (Jacoby 1984, p.118). This may happen at a wider than personal level: before and during the Second World War, the Nazis projected their own unconscious shadow qualities, which they rejected, onto the Jews and scapegoated them accordingly. Transference and countertransference are particular cases of projection in the therapeutic relationship.

TRANSFERENCE

Freud was the first to describe this phenomenon in which the client's 'un-satisfied or repressed wishes of the past tend to get transferred to a new object, namely the analyst' (Jacoby 1984, p.15). He felt that transference was a necessary part of the therapeutic process in order to discover its cause. Whenever we say that a counsellor or other clinical professional reminds us of another person, that is transference; we may not even be aware that we are doing this. Thus a client may unconsciously behave towards her counsellor as if he were her overbearing father. One patient I worked with named me Doctor Death; in that way, his unbearable feelings about his terminal illness were transferred onto me.

COUNTERTRANSFERENCE

This is the therapist's transference onto the client (Jacoby 1984, p.38). It may be concordant, where the therapist's feeling response is empathically in concord with the client, or complementary, where the therapist's response takes the opposite pole to that of the client; thus, feeling like a critical maternal figure in response to the client's withdrawn adolescent behaviour. In the past, it was felt that countertransference got in the way of therapy. Now, it is seen as a helpful part of the therapeutic process. The counsellor's feeling reaction to the client may actually give useful information about him. Thus, if the therapist feels judgemental about the client, this may reflect the client tending to behave like a victim in his relationships.

EMOTIONS AND FEELINGS

These terms are often used interchangeably (Freshwater and Robertson 2002). Emotion may be thought of as the physiological process, say of fear or anger – the bodily changes that occur, the increased heart rate, dilated pupils and so on. It does not necessarily imply consciousness. It is possible to react to a threat pre-consciously. This is presumably the state that animals experience, as when a rabbit is hunted by a fox.

Feelings, however, imply an awareness of the emotional state. They are complex because a particular emotion will be associated with multiple past memories which go to making up the feeling state. Expression is more sophisticated, too. We can give words to our sorrow. This is how Marie Cardinal (1993, p.10) described her distress in the book she wrote about her analysis:

> Curled up like a ball, heels against buttocks, arms holding the knees, strong, tight against the chest, nails dug so deep into the palms of her hands they eventually pierced her skin, her head rocking back and forth or side to side, feeling so heavy, the blood and sweat was pouring out of her. The Thing, which on the inside was made of a monstrous crawling of images, sounds, and odours, projected in every way by a devastating pulse making all reasoning incoherent, all explanation absurd, all efforts to order tentative and useless, was revealed on the outside by violent shaking and nauseating sweat.

HEALING AND CURING

'Cure' means eradication of an illness. By definition, this is not a feature of the physical aspects of palliative care. Healing, however, is different. While it can have the same sense as curing, it means more. Its Old English root, *haelen*, is also the origin of the words 'whole', 'holy' and 'hale'. They point to a state of being where a person is in harmony with himself and those around him, is in a state of homeostasis internally and relatedness externally. This may happen with the dying, as they face what is, in the end, a natural and universal process.

An old man, originally from Cyprus, was close to death. He had become estranged from his sons and had not seen them for years. He didn't even have their addresses. He was adamant that he wanted to see them before he died. At times it seemed he was within hours of dying but he hung on to life and the days passed. The hospice was able to trace one son who came to visit him. It was a deeply felt reunion. We thought he would die then but still he clung to life. A few days later his other son was found and he, too, came to see him. He died the next day. His life had been out of balance, in the rift in his relationship with his children. His healing reunion with them allowed him to die peacefully.

CHAPTER 2

Meeting

THE SETTING

The usual counselling setting is of a room with chairs for the counsellor and client. In palliative care the setting is much more diverse. Many patients have single rooms, but they may be in a three- or four-bedded bay, in which case the other patients and their visiting family might be listening with fascination to the discussion. Obviously confidentiality is compromised, and yet patients are often too ill to move from their beds to talk in a private room. Having the curtains drawn does provide a *feeling* of privacy and patients are usually able to talk personally in this context. This approach, admittedly less than ideal, works better than might be expected. Other settings include counselling and out-patient rooms, the hospice garden, the sitting room or seeing the patient at home. Nurses I've worked with tell me that patients sometimes talk more openly about their feelings when they are being given a bath: their physical nakedness and vulnerability facilitates an emotional openness.

FIRST IMPRESSIONS

These start from the moment that you hear anything about the patient, such as his clinical history, even before you have set eyes on him. So often, staff have said to me that this patient is difficult, or that one is delightful, and already I am forming an image of them which may be biased. When you actually meet the patient, first impressions are particularly important because your preconceptions about the patient are still relatively few and you see them with fresh eyes and hear them with fresh ears. These are, in fact, your first countertransference reactions and less likely to be affected by the urge to suppress uncomfortable feelings or thoughts. They will not tell you everything about a patient – how could they? They will tell you something about her persona, that is the way she presents herself to the world. Part of this will be the way she does or does not interact with her family and whether she talks or a family member takes over as spokesperson, re-enacting a long-held family pattern. In this situation, it may be necessary to insist, at times against opposition, that you hear the story directly from the patient rather than by proxy.

We need to ask ourselves, too, what impressions we are making on the patient and his family. People who work in the healing professions do so at the interface between life and death, hope and despair. It is not surprising, then, that they are the subject of multifarious projections (Heyse-Moore 2007). Table 2.1 sets out some of the ways clinicians are viewed, albeit unconsciously. Many of these are transferable between disciplines.

Table 2.1 Some ways that clinicians are perceived by patients

DOCTOR	NURSE	SOCIAL WORKER	MINISTER
Healer	Angel	Counsellor	Priest
Pharmacologist	Mother (good and bad)	Listener	Magician
Miracle worker		Parent	Miracle worker
Symptomatologist	Carer	Advocate	Prophet
Surgeon	Supporter	Family supporter	God's messenger
Diagnostician	Listener	Lady almoner	Judas/betrayer
Scientist	Comforter	House hunter	Inquisitor
Experimenter	Friend	Grant provider	Judge
Doctor Death	Attractive	Child snatcher	Scapegoat
Butcher	Guide		
Quack	Controlling		
Cold	Enabler		

Patients, then, will be studying you very carefully, taking in how you're dressed, how you behave and how you talk. Consider that when you're getting dressed in the morning and look in your mirror. While they will be looking for someone who is competent, they will, perhaps even more, be looking for someone who understands and is sympathetic to their problems.

ON SITTING DOWN

When I was a house surgeon, I, along with other doctors and a gaggle of medical students, followed my eminent consultant around the ward. He would talk at length with us or quiz the students and then, standing at the foot of the bed, say a few words to the patient. This is such a common sight, even now, that it is little remarked on. And yet, to stand over a person lying in bed sends a signal: I am superior to you. Patients are already feeling exposed – they have been divested of their clothes along with their health and may well have become parted from their teeth and their glasses too. It is doubly important, therefore, as far as is possible to meet them on equal terms and to respect their vulnerability. Sitting with a patient means you are at about eye level – on a par therefore. It implies you're giving them time, time to talk – standing can suggest hurriedness and the wish to move on.

In the Victoria and Albert Museum, there is a little wooden figurine of a Japanese nobleman. He is seated in the lotus position, meditating. He has a tall hat and his robes flow to the ground forming a triangle, like a mountain. It is no coincidence that, in Buddhism, this posture is associated with the mountain and its strength, solidity and stability. It isn't necessary to be Buddhist to see that these sitting qualities will impart a sense of safety to the patient.

At home, you will only allow onto your bed those you are close to – your partner or your children, for example. It is an intimate space. For this reason, if there isn't a chair available, it is important always to ask permission of a patient to sit on his bed.

Of course, it's not always about sitting. I remember coming across a relative in crisis who was crouched down in the hospice corridor by some swing doors. The first thing I did was to crouch alongside her, a form of physical mirroring, I suppose.

RELATIONSHIP

I recently came across the words of a headstone inscription from a Canadian graveyard that said: 'Here lies George Brown, born a man, died a gastroenterologist' (Remen 1997, p.42). I laughed when I read this, but it was poignant too. Unintentionally, it pointed to a common dilemma particularly affecting doctors, but also other clinical disciplines: can I be myself, a person, with sick people or must I be subsumed by my role? My contention is that both are important.

Martin Buber, the Hasidic Jewish philosopher, wrote an important and influential book, *I and Thou* (1958). In it he distinguished two forms of relating, I–Thou, and I–It. By I–Thou, he meant relating in depth, person to person, where we can say we have truly met another person. By I–It, he meant relationships which treat the other, whether human or inanimate, as a separate object. Both may occur in a conversation. This is not to criticise I–It relating. It is a necessary part of everyday functioning. Our medical or nursing or social work roles require it. Patients expect their clinicians to be competent. But they want them to be people too. So, an interweaving of these two strands of relating is needed. A musical analogy may be useful here. Music needs structure – an agreed method of writing it down, rules of composition, types of instrument and so on. But, all of these carry the actual music, the sound of the muse that can transport us in a moment, without which the structure is an empty skeleton. To take this metaphor further, two different melodies may interweave harmoniously in a composition, a good image for conversation in depth.

Althea

I invited Althea into the out-patients room where her community nurse specialist, Sue, was also waiting. I could see Althea was nervous, breathing fast. She was expensively but quietly dressed and her long blonde hair had been skilfully highlighted and carefully brushed. Her make-up was subtle. She was wearing perfume. All of this despite having two young children. My impression was that she had taken a lot of care with her appearance preparing for this visit, almost like one would for an examination. I noted the unconscious pun I had made on educational and clinical examination. She seemed to be making a statement about her femininity, her attractiveness, despite her illness. When we shook hands, I noticed her palms were cold and sweating. I invited her to sit down and felt her staring anxiously at me. One of her stockings had a small ladder in it – rather like an Achilles heel I thought ruefully. I felt a wish to reassure her, and yet knew, from my previous discussions with Sue that Althea's bone metastases had spread and were causing her pain; hence the visit.

Note in the above example how quickly a complex array of impressions are picked up in the first few moments of meeting.

CHAPTER 3

Attending Skills

Giving another person your undivided attention is both powerful and healing. What do I mean by this? Take this description of how Freud gave attention, as an example:

> It struck me so forcibly that I shall never forget him. He had qualities which I had never seen in any other man. Never had I seen such concentrated attention. There was none of the piercing 'soul penetrating gaze' business. His eyes were mild and genial. His voice was low and kind. His gestures were few. But the attention he gave me, his appreciation of what I said, even when I said it badly, was extraordinary. You've no idea what it meant to be listened to like that. (Carnegie 1988, p.106)

We have all experienced this, and know its value. To highlight this point, consider the opposite, what happens when attention is withheld. This was the experience of Jean-Dominique Bauby (1998, p.61) a man with the locked-in syndrome whose only remaining voluntary movements were to be able to nod his head and blink his left eye. He awoke one morning to find the hospital ophthalmologist sewing his right eyelid shut. Bauby was terrified that the doctor might sew his other eyelid shut, too, thus depriving him of blinking as his only means of communicating with the outside world. He tried to signal questions to the doctor, who took no notice of him – an irony since he specialised in eyes. Bauby wrote with much feeling about this uncaring, disdainful specialist, his abruptness and his caustic manner. I wonder myself whether the doctor ever read this evaluation of his bedside manner – it would have been an example of seeing ourselves as others see us.

How, then, can we give attention effectively ourselves? First we must look at where our attention is directed. It needs to be both outwards, to the patient, and inwards, to our own inner process. Table 3.1 lists some of the ways we can do this. Just hearing the patient's words is not enough. We need to attend with all our senses and inner awareness.

Table 3.1 Modes of attention

ATTENTION	TYPE
Outer awareness	Listening
	Observing
	Body language
	Touch
	Smell
Inner awareness	Mind
	Feelings
	Body
	Intuition
Process	Stories and meanings

OUTER ATTENTION
Listening

Here is how Herman Hesse described this skill in his book *Siddhartha*:

> Later, when the sun was beginning to set, they sat on a tree trunk by the river and Siddhartha told him about his origin and his life and how he had seen him today after that hour of despair. The story lasted late into the night. Vasudeva listened with great attention; he heard all about his origin and childhood, about his studies, his seekings, his pleasures and needs. It was one of the ferryman's greatest virtues that, like few people, he knew how to listen. Without his saying a word, the speaker felt that Vasudeva took in every word, quietly, expectantly, that he missed nothing. He did not await anything with impatience and gave neither praise nor blame – he only listened. Siddhartha felt how wonderful it was to have such a listener, who could be absorbed in his own life, his own strivings, his own sorrows. (Hesse 1991, pp.83–4, first published 1922)

Here, then, are some essential elements to good listening: focus, unhurriedness, interest and avoidance of judgement. Note that the focusing will not only be on the story, but the way it is told. Here are some scenarios as examples:

- He spoke slowly, formally and precisely, correcting the doctor if she didn't understand the point he was making.
- Words tumbled from her in a disordered, passionate stream.
- He spoke slowly with some effort and a strong, Eastern European accent.
- When she started talking about her illness, she became hesitant and avoided the word cancer.
- He assured the doctor, as if passing the time of day, that he had come to terms with his illness.
- She could scarcely speak in between the sobs.
- Angry invective poured from him as he bitterly criticised the hospital doctors for not diagnosing his wife's cancer soon enough.
- In her confusion, she had reverted to her native Italian tongue.

Observing

All clinicians are trained to observe in ways consonant with their discipline. Doctors examine the body diagnostically; nurses might focus on pressure sores or mobility; social workers look for clues to their client's emotional state or social behaviour. However, we can always learn more. Here is an example from the experience of an American physician which included observation through sight, touch and smell: There was an announcement at his hospital that Yeshi Dhonden, personal physician to the Dalai Lama, would be making rounds and would examine a patient whose diagnosis he did not know. He had begun the day early by bathing, fasting and prayer. Watched by a group of suspicious Western physicians, he first observed the woman he had been asked to see. There were no apparent signs of disease. He took her pulse.

> For the next half-hour he remains thus, suspended above the patient like some exotic golden bird. All the power of the man seems to have

been drawn into this one purpose. It is palpation of the pulse raised to the state of ritual.

Then he examined her urine by whipping it into a foam with sticks and inhaling the odour. In the conference room he spoke of:

> winds coursing through the body of the woman, currents that break against barriers eddying. These vortices are in her blood, the last spending of an imperfect heart. Between the chambers of the heart, long, long before she was born, a wind had come and blown open a deep gate that must never be opened. Through it charge the full waters of her river, as the mountain stream cascades in springtime, battering, knocking loose the land and flooding her breath.

The diagnosis is then revealed in Western terms: interventricular septal defect due to congenital heart disease and resultant cardiac failure. His was a poetic yet exact description of this pathology (Dass and Gorman 1986, pp.117–21). So, even when we simply look at a patient, there may be much more to see than at first meets the eye. This observing is not only clinical but also personal. What does it tell us about the human being before us? The psychotherapist Thomas Moore (1994 p.155) has this to say:

> The human body is an immense source of imagination, a field on which imagination plays wantonly. The body is the soul presented in its richest and most expressive form. In the body, we see the soul articulated in gesture, dress, movement, shape, physiognomy, temperature, skin eruptions, tics, diseases – in countless expressive forms.

Next time you see a patient, try putting this into practice. Here are some examples:

- What is it like for a woman to wear a wig because she is bald from chemotherapy?
- Why is this man expressionless and looking down at the floor as he talks to me?
- Is she wearing a high collar to hide the swelling lymph nodes in her neck?
- How come he is so restless and keeps getting up to pace the room?
- She is lying curled up in bed in a foetal position. What is the message here?

- There's a half-empty bottle of whisky on the bed-side locker and he is draining his glass.

- She is reading a book on alternative therapies for curing cancer.

- As soon as he starts talking about his cancer, his wife gets up and leaves the room.

- Her seven-year-old son plays with his toys in the corner of the room, seemingly oblivious of her conversation with the doctor about her illness.

Body language

It's clear from the above examples that patients speak to us through their bodies as much as through words, though they may not be aware of doing so. This is not static; rather, their communication is changing all the time through gestures and expressions. We are all experts at interpreting this language; we've learnt to do so since birth. In fact, it goes beyond this – we pick up signals instinctively. Body language evolved in early humans long before speech and is, therefore, deeply ingrained in the ancestral pre-conscious portions of our brains, the prime-itive domain of instinct and emotions, and of the fight, flight or freeze responses to threat. No wonder, then, that we can have an uncomfortable feeling about a patient but not know why.

I remember one patient who had advanced abdominal cancer. He was in his forties and had suffered brain damage following a head injury many years ago, since when he had not spoken, although he appeared to comprehend some words. The only way to understand *him* was through his body. If he felt hungry, he would take an apple from another patient's locker. If he felt low, he would lie curled up in bed, his face to the wall. If he felt frightened he would put his hands over his ears and shake his head. His experience was immediate, in the here and now. A mental understanding of his cancer and its consequences was not in his ambit, and, in this way, he was apparently spared the anxieties of wondering what the future would bring. Interestingly, this has resonances with the Buddhist practice of being present in the moment, since the past has gone and the future is yet to materialise.

Some body language may be obvious. Crossed legs and folded arms suggest defendedness; constant jiggling of a foot points to anxiety;

flushing to embarrassment. Patients may cover their eyes or ears as if to say, I can't bear to see, or hear, this. They may touch the painful area or keep their hands on it protectively. Or, they may place their hand on their heart if moved to tears. Some signals are more subtle: faster breathing, variations in pupil size or grinding of teeth are examples.

One way that patients communicate is through tears. A common reflex here is to pass them the tissues box. However, this can give a message that it's not all right to cry, which can halt their inner process. It is better to watch and wait; when there is a natural pause, or if the patient requests it, then pass them the tissues.

Touch

An initial handshake is a useful and socially sanctioned way of making contact with a patient on a human level. It suggests equality and cooperation and may help to reduce anxiety at meeting the clinician. The actual handshake gives messages, such as the strong but trembling handshake of an emaciated, terminally ill man that says: I'm struggling to stay in charge. Some patients miss your hand because they've had a stroke; some are blind so that you have to pick their hand up; and there is the cold, clammy handshake of fear.

Doctors are in the privileged position of being allowed to examine patients, and nurses to attend to their bodily needs, so involving physical contact. While this is primarily for clinical reasons, it also tells us something about the individual. For example:

- She won't let herself be examined.
- He holds his abdomen tense during palpation.
- She has not been looking after her colostomy bag leaving the skin sore.
- He has advanced lung cancer and his fingers are still stained with nicotine.
- She has needle puncture marks in her arm from her long-term heroin use.
- Tattooed on his forearm is the number he was assigned in his concentration camp during the Second World War.

- She has a large, fungating breast cancer which she has ignored for many years.

Examination is, however, not just observational. You communicate your attitude to the patient through touch just as much as you do with words. I remember, as a medical student, seeing a consultant examine the abdomen of a patient with pancreatic cancer so forcefully that she was left in serious pain afterwards. Conversely, you can communicate respect, gentleness, strength, skill, interest and unhurriedness. Touch has an intimate and calming quality which is utilised in massage. A clinical examination or nursing procedure can, then, also be therapeutic, can be healing. Dr Rachel Naomi Remen (1997, pp.238–40) describes an interesting example of this. Part of a workshop she teaches for doctors involves the therapeutic effect of touch, 'hands-on healing' as she calls it, a departure from the way doctors usually touch patients, though more familiar, perhaps, to nurses. She comments: 'while it is a great privilege to do this with people with cancer, watching physicians heal each other is one of the most moving things I have witnessed anywhere.' They seem to have 'a deep and intuitive knowledge of each other's wounds'. One doctor had gone through a divorce; he localised the pain of it in his heart. He described how his companion, a surgeon, placed her hand on his chest. 'I was really astonished by how warm her hand was, and how gently and tenderly she touched me…the warmth of her hand seemed to…surround my heart…it seemed to me as if she was holding my heart in her hand… I felt the strength of her hand, how rock-steady she was…'

Smell

Does this seem an unimportant sense when we give attention to another person? It, too, has its place:

- The man who smells of alcohol at 9 am. How did he become alcoholic?
- The shame of the woman who smells of urine but denies incontinence.
- The unwashed smell of the man admitted because of self-neglect. Why did he give up taking care of himself?
- The woman who always wears perfume and then, one day, stops. Why?

INNER ATTENTION
Thinking

Carl Rogers (1961, p.18) had this to say about understanding:

> I have found it of enormous value when I can permit myself to understand another person. The way in which I have worded this statement may seem strange to you. Is it necessary to permit oneself to understand another? I think that it is. Our first reaction to most of the statements which we hear from other people is an immediate evaluation, or judgement, rather than an understanding of it. When someone expresses some feeling or attitude or belief, our tendency is, almost immediately, to feel 'That's right'; or 'That's stupid'; 'That's abnormal'; 'That's unreasonable'; 'That's incorrect'; 'That's not nice.' Very rarely do we permit ourselves to understand precisely what the meaning of the statement is to him. I believe this is because understanding is risky. If I let myself really understand another person, I might be changed by that understanding. And we all fear change. So as I say, it is not an easy thing to permit ourselves to understand an individual, to enter thoroughly and completely and empathically into his frame of reference. It is also a rare thing.

Much thinking in health care is clinician-centred – how can *I* solve this problem for the patient? While this is obviously important, Rogers is inviting us to step out of this mould and, as the saying goes, into the patient's shoes (or even slippers). We have all experienced this happening to us at some time, and it is very potent. The listener seems, empathically, to know you. This relates back to early childhood. One of the essential aspects of the mother–baby relationship is that she mirrors what happens with her child, she connects empathically with his feeling state and communicates this, whether by expression, words or tone of voice. Babies need this experience. Lacking it, they are vulnerable to severe emotional disturbances. No wonder, then, that we respond to empathy in such a visceral way (Winnicott 1988).

Understanding does not always come easy. One elderly, dying patient I looked after had systematically abused his daughter sexually over many years. He showed no signs of regretting what he had done and she, still under his sway though he was so ill, visited regularly and submissively. Why trouble to understand someone like that who has behaved so destructively? Who would want to enter his frame of reference? Aside from the professional duty of care, there is a crucial difference between understanding and condoning. Had we been able to investigate this man's appalling behaviour, we might have discovered uncomfortable truths – he, too, may have been abused as a child, might once have been a victim – as happens all too commonly. This does nothing to excuse his behaviour, but does offer an insight into his motivation, a clearer perspective than blind condemnation.

Feelings

It is inevitable you will have feeling reactions to patients. It is worth paying attention to these countertransferences. They may tell you something useful. If you feel sad or irritated, it is possible you are picking up these feelings from the patient even if he himself has repressed his emotions. A simple comment such as: 'How are you feeling?' or: 'You seem a bit sad at the moment', can then help him to get in touch with his rejected feelings and what their message is.

One form of this is projective identification, (Jacobs 1998, p.53) a remarkable phenomenon first described by the psychoanalyst Melanie Klein. An example of this occurred when I was talking with a relative who was calmly telling me that she was going to commit suicide when her partner died. After we left the meeting, the doctor who was accompanying me experienced intense feelings of nausea and despair, something he had not been feeling before the discussion. What had happened? The relative had, as it were, projected her unbearably painful feelings of despair onto this doctor, who had taken them in, was identifying with them and was experiencing them for her. This strange process is a widely described occurrence in therapy. There are three points to draw from this. First, be aware that this can happen and that the feelings experienced are not your own. If you don't recognise this, you may be left wondering where in your own psyche these intense emotions came from. Second, having identified this process, it is possible to put this back to the patient or relative. For example: 'I imagine you may be having feelings that are difficult to let in because they're so painful.' Third, take some time after such a meeting to let go of any feelings you are still carrying, for example by talking with a colleague.

Is it appropriate to share your feelings with patients? The key questions here are: What will be helpful and relevant to them? And when? Usually it is possible to get a sense of what works for them. It depends too, of course, on the rapport that has developed between you. Some patients appreciate this fellow feeling as part of the empathetic bond between you and it helps them in their inner process. Thus: 'I felt sad when you told me about your loss.' They sense you are relating to them person to person, not just in a clinician's role. For others, it is not appropriate. They want you to be the competent doctor or professional nurse with the answers and they don't wish to see you in another light. This flexible approach differs from the traditional attitude of a dispassionate clinical demeanour, where feelings hardly enter the equation. It is, however, possible to demonstrate both competence and care in relating to patients.

Sometimes, when you see a patient you are already experiencing feelings related to your own life, such as sadness because a close friend has died or anger at a difficult colleague. These are important, but, during the encounter with the patient, they need to be 'bracketed', kept contained for the moment in order to give your full attention to the ill person. Later, when you have time for yourself, you can return to them and give them the consideration they need. This is about taking a professional approach to your work. If your feelings are so overwhelming that you can't bracket them, then it's better to take some time out, which might include talking to a colleague or supervisor, until their intensity has become manageable. This approach is different from repression of feelings into the unconscious in a stern attempt to stay in control.

Body

Any thought, feeling or perception that you experience will affect your body. If you feel threatened, your pulse and breathing will accelerate and your pupils dilate. If you feel sad, tears may form in your eyes, you may sob and your voice may become choked. If you're not in touch with how you feel, scan your body. Notice any sensations and focus on them. You may then find that they amplify into a feeling state. A heaviness in the chest may be a precursor to sadness; restlessness may signal incipient anger. The body never lies.

Common bodily reactions in staff include headache, tiredness or sleepiness. While it would not be surprising for tired nurses or exhausted doctors to experience these through lack of sleep or overwork, they can also indicate what's happening with the patient:

- *Headache*: the anxious patient who talks so fast you can't take it all in.

- *Tiredness*: talking with a melancholic patient.

- *Sleepiness*: this can signal that a feeling state is being unconsciously repressed because it is too painful or too threatening to the patient.

Intuition

Despite their scientific training, even doctors will use phrases such as: 'My gut feeling about this is...' or: 'This doesn't feel right' or: 'I can't put my finger on it, but...' or: 'I have a hunch about this', in their everyday work. Other clinical disciplines may be less inhibited in this respect. I always took note if a nurse told me that a patient didn't look right though she couldn't say why. Such hunches often turned out to be right. Some nurses I worked with even knew in advance when a patient would die. In practice, then, we give some regard to our intuitive reactions even if objective evidence is lacking. I believe it makes sense to treat intuitions as hypotheses to be tested – some turn out to fit, some don't, but to ignore them completely would be to miss a potentially valuable source of understanding.

We have already touched on the polarities of brain function – of rationality on the one hand and imagery, emotions and understanding wholes on the other, and their complex relationship to left and right brain activity. One view of intuitions is that they occur when the psychological activity initially mediated by the right cerebral hemisphere grasps a situation just ahead of its rational left-sided partner, or is temporarily dominant over it. At such moments, consciousness is mediated by a comprehension of wholes, of feelings and visual impressions – in other words, an intuitive mode of perception. This, then, is a way of processing observations which is just as important as, and complements, the analytic approach originating in the left brain, the two synthesising to provide a fuller perception than either separately (Carter 1999, p.40). Others argue that intuition is a transpersonal quality, an emanation of the higher unconscious (see Chapter 5).

PROCESS
Narratives and meanings

Every clinician has met the patient who talks at inordinate length about her illness, rehearsing every detail, repeating herself, providing a mass of clinically irrelevant information. While this is frustrating for the clinician, there is another way of looking at what is happening. The patient is telling a story, the story of her illness, and it's important to her that she does so.

Stories are a part of all human cultures and they serve a deep need: to make sense of our lives, to discover a meaning in them. This is what patients are trying to do when they recount the narrative of their illnesses. Why is this important? We need meaning in our lives in the same way as we need air to breathe – it is like the golden thread that guides us through the labyrinthine twists and turns of life. It is the person plunged in meaninglessness who is in crisis.

This need was demonstrated by Victor Frankl (2004, first published 1946), a concentration camp inmate during the Second World War. He was a psychotherapist and he knew the dangers of lapsing into despair in this extreme situation. As a survival strategy, he studied the behaviour of the camp guards and prisoners from the perspective of his profession. He noticed that those inmates with a sense of purpose in their lives were more likely to survive than those who did not. He worked as a doctor supporting traumatised prisoners and organised a suicide watch unit. For himself, he kept the memories and images of being with his wife before the war alive by constantly thinking of her. His aim was to see her again after the war. He did survive, though his wife died in another concentration camp. He later created a new form of psychological therapy – logotherapy – based on meaning.

This, then, is not just a neat idea; it can keep us alive. For the dying, this may not apply physically, but it does psychologically and spiritually. Many people really do live their dying, and will say that they have felt far more alive during their illness than before when they were well. Their priorities have shifted to what and who is important to them in their lives

Patients will work out their own understanding of their illness. Some will want an orthodox medical explanation as to how their cancer arose. A woman may decide, however, that the cause of her breast cancer was an injury to the area of the breast containing the cancer that she sustained six months before her diagnosis, even though the cancer would have begun long before then. Similarly, a man may feel that his brain tumour relates to a fractured skull he had after a car accident. Patients may hold to their sometimes idiosyncratic views even if such opinions don't tally with the clinical facts. One way of understanding such events is that they represent what Jung called 'synchronicity' (Storr 1998, pp.339–41), a puzzling phenomenon whereby two events occur at the same time which are meaningfully linked but not causally connected. A familiar example is when we find ourselves thinking about a friend we have not seen for a year and that friend phones minutes later. Jung mentions the example of a woman who remembered birds gathering outside the windows of the death-chamber of her mother and grandmother when they died. Years later, her husband collapsed in the street and was brought home dying. She was, however, already acutely anxious before she knew of his crisis because a flock of birds had alighted on the house (at the time he became ill) and she feared a death was imminent, as turned out to be the case.

While it's important to respect patients' views, there is one area where it may be necessary to challenge their understanding. This is if they see their cancer as their fault, or a punishment. Thus, one elderly woman was fearful and guilt-ridden on admission to a hospice. After she had got to know and trust the staff, she confided tearfully to one of them that she had had an illegitimate child as a teenager. To her, her gynaecological cancer was a punishment for this, as she saw it, shameful secret. Clearly here it was important to work with her on forgiving herself. A key part of this was for her to see that the staff she talked to did not judge her, but rather accepted and respected her just as she was.

Clinicians have a long tradition of telling stories, recognising their importance. Medical authors include Arthur Conan Doyle, Somerset Maugham and Chekhov. Dame Cicely Saunders, who was by turns a social worker, nurse and doctor, often wrote about the dying patients she cared for. Furthermore, illness and dying are frequent subjects of novels, poems, plays or personal accounts. Shakespeare's *Hamlet* addresses the themes of depression and suicide. The Greek myth of Chiron the centaur, who was struck by a poisonous arrow, focuses on the incurable wound. Dylan Thomas' poem, 'Do not go gentle into that good night', speaks to the rage of the dying. Here we can see the use of metaphors to provide a container for the inarticulate rawness of dying. One thing we can do, then, is to help patients find their own metaphors for the story of their illness.

Jean-Dominique Bauby, who had a massive stroke, leaving him paralysed apart from being able to blink one eyelid, did this by writing a book of stories about his illness. How? Through using a system of blinks to communicate words and letters to a scribe. In this extraordinarily laborious way the book was completed. He called it *The Diving Bell and the Butterfly*. The diving bell was his image for his paralysed body, and the butterfly represented his mind taking flight. Movingly, he describes how he was able to let his imagination roam freely where it would – to far lands, into the stories of history and myths, to visit those he loved and to remember his childhood. He wrote with a poet's eye about the small events of his daily life – a visit from his speech therapist, a wheelchair promenade, painstaking attempts to communicate with visitors. He died shortly after completing the book (Bauby 1998).

CHAPTER 4

Core Counselling Skills

There may be a temptation to think of counselling skills as magic keys to unlock the inner workings of a patient's mind. Or to treat them as if they are weapons: if they are not working, add more, bring on the heavy artillery. Actually, the dictum: 'Less is more' is nearer the truth. To illustrate this, here is a story about Carl Rogers, who founded person-centred therapy, giving a demonstration session to a group of doctors (Remen 1997, pp.218–19):

> Rogers conducted it without saying a single word, conveying to his client simply by the quality of his attention a total acceptance of him exactly as he was. The doctor began to talk and the session rapidly became a great deal more than the demonstration of a technique. In the safe climate of Rogers's total acceptance, he began to shed his masks, hesitantly at first and then more and more easily. As each mask fell, Rogers welcomed the one behind it unconditionally...

Perhaps, then, it is better to see them as useful tools, adjuncts to the developing relationship between client and therapist, between patient and clinician.

In the discussion that follows, remember that about 7 per cent of communication is content, 38 per cent relates to tone and 55 per cent is non-verbal (Bayliss 2004, p.67). Your words alone are not enough. It is the way you say them and your body language that make the greater impression.

REFLECTIVE SKILLS

These are used for 'capturing what clients are telling you and repeating the message in your own words' (Culley and Bond 2004, p.18). They include restating, paraphrasing and summarising. They all mirror back to the patient what he has just said. I have also included affirmative responses such as 'mmm', which are a part of any conversation. While they are simple, they are powerful interventions, referring back as they do to the primal mirroring relationship between mother and child already referred to (Winnicott 1988). The following dialogue illustrates how they might be used.

Althea transcript

Althea: The thing is, well, I just feel scared of where the cancer will strike next.

Louis: Where it will strike next? [*restating*]

Althea: Yes, I mean I know it's in my spine and I'm worried it will spread to other bones...

Louis: Mmm.

Althea: That would be such a disaster...[begins to cry]... I can't afford to get any iller. I've got two young children to look after, and they're a handful – Jack has been waking a lot at night and crying for me.

Louis: [nods head]

Althea: And my husband's away often, he gets tired, so I can't expect him to be their main carer as well...and there's my teaching job. We need the money; they've been very good about my taking time off but there is a limit...

Louis: So...we're looking at your worries about getting iller...and the effect it might have on your life; on your children and your husband...

Althea: Yes.

Louis: ...and also on your job and your finances. [*summarising*]

Althea: That's right; it's too awful to think about, but I have to, especially for my family's sake. I don't want them to have to suffer because of me.

Louis: Althea, I'm very aware of your deep concern to take care of and protect your family. [*paraphrasing*]

Affirmative responses

We all use some form of this response when listening to others. It's a way of saying: I'm listening to you. Responses, as well as mmm, might include uh-huh, yes, sure, OK and so on. Usually this is with a nod of the head to emphasise understanding of what's been said. Furthermore, you can convey a wide range of feelings just by saying mmm: empathy, sadness, humour, fear and questioning for example. Like all good things, you can have too much of it. An over-eager 'mmm' with an over-emphatic nodding of the head can put the patient off.

Restating

Here, the last few words, or word, that the patient has just said are repeated, especially if they have paused. It's a way of helping them to continue their reflections. It needs to be employed judiciously. Used mechanically, it can sound like parroting. One way of preventing this is to change the inflection slightly, giving it a questioning tone as in the example above.

Paraphrasing

This is a restatement of what the patient said in different words. While it is another way of empathising with the patient, the difference in wording implies you have taken in what she has said and reflected on it. It implies you have listened to her seriously. Sometimes, too, patients are inarticulate or ramble and a clear paraphrase can help them understand better what they're trying to say.

Summarising

Summaries are useful in a number of ways (Culley and Bond 2004, pp.38–9):

- to clarify what the patient has said and what she is feeling
- to review the discussion so far
- to end a discussion
- as a way of beginning another meeting where it was agreed beforehand what the starting agenda will be
- to help clients prioritise what the most important issues are for them

- to help move the process of the session forward. This can be done first by forming a choice point, as in the following dialogue:

Althea transcript

Louis: Althea, we've looked at some of the issues that are troubling you, your concerns about the spread of the cancer in your spine, and of the effects on your family and your work. Is there one of these that you would like to focus on first?

Althea: I suppose it's what's happening with the cancer. I'm so worried about what it might do to me.

The other way of moving the process forward is by employing a figure-ground perspective. This makes use of an artistic analogy – in a painting the main figure stands out while the other parts fade into the background. So it is with a patient's concerns. Often, one issue will stand out; the others are still there, but more as a backdrop to the main theme. This means listening to the patient's narrative and picking out what is the theme she is most concerned with, most often returns to, and then checking with her if she wishes to focus on this for the session. The figure may change over time. Frequently, when, say, a patient's anxiety recedes, then depression or sadness takes over as the foreground complaint. Interestingly, this can happen with physical symptoms too. When the pain in one area is controlled, then another pain or a different symptom such as breathlessness may present itself. A game of 'Chase the Symptom' may ensue. It's as though there is an underlying suffering which expresses itself through different physical or psychological symptoms.

EXPLORATORY SKILLS

While reflective skills are essential in counselling, their use means that the content of the client's narrative rests with him. It is also important to use exploratory skills. Here, the therapist takes a more active, enquiring role, bringing in his perspective on the content being discussed. This means entering the client's inner world and investigating it with her. This is her private space. We enter only with her agreement. To do otherwise would be intrusive.

It is important to strike a balance between these two approaches. In practice, their use will mean a constant shifting between their perspectives during one conversation. Breaking bad news, for example, by its very nature is exploratory, but it requires an empathic, supportive approach too as the feelings associated with the discovery of a serious illness surface. A purely reflective approach can run the risk of endless recirculation of the same material. An overly exploratory line may feel persecutory and cause the patient to close up to protect himself.

Two exploratory methods will be considered – questions and statements.

Questions

These are the stock in trade of doctors and nurses: 'Where is your pain?' 'How many hours a night do you sleep?' 'How long have you been breath-less?' 'How often are you sick?' and so on. An endless list of factual questions, which patients expect and usually cooperate with. Even psycho-logical symptoms get the same treatment: 'How long have you felt anxious?' 'How severe is the depression?' This approach derives from the paradigm of the body as a machine. Practitioners are skilled in diagnosis and treatment, technicians in control. The patient is relatively passive.

But questions in counselling have a different purpose. They are about the client's self-discovery, about him finding his own answers. Yes, we can give a patient information about the state of his cancer, but we are also there to assist him with his feelings about his illness and in deciding for himself what action to take. Very often it will be conventional – 'Yes, I'll have the chemotherapy'. But, there may be surprises. He may elect not to have life-saving treatment. He may decide to put his faith in unproven complementary therapies. While clinicians have a responsibility to give the patient the facts about treatment, it may equally be important to explore with him his feelings about taking the path he has chosen. Perhaps he doesn't want treatment because he wants to be with his wife who died recently. Doctors will sometimes try to make a reluctant patient have the 'correct' treatment. Actually, we have no right to do this. Perhaps the energy so invested would be better employed in understanding his point of view. He might then be more prepared to consider what the clinician has to say. It is like Aesop's fable in which the sun and the wind vied with each other to get the coat off a traveller's back. The wind blew as hard as he was able but the traveller simply pulled his coat more tightly around him. The sun shone gently and as the man grew warmer, he took off his coat of his own accord.

Rudyard Kipling (1902) wrote a poem about his six honest serving men: What, Why, When, How, Where and Who. We shall see that these have different functions in counselling as compared with taking a clinical history.

Closed and open questions

Closed questions include those that require a yes or no answer or a brief factual response such as your age, job and so on. While useful for information gathering, they don't invite self-exploration. Questions such as: 'Do you feel anxious when you wake up in the morning?' can shut the conversational door. 'What makes you anxious?' however, which is an open question, invites a broad reply.

Kipling's six honest serving men can give us some pointers to using open questions:

- What does it feel like to have cancer?
- When do you find you get depressed?
- How do you get into arguments with your partner?
- Where in your body do you experience the sadness?
- Who supports you when you feel upset?

The 'why?' question has not been included for a number of reasons. First, it may put pressure on the patient to justify herself. Second, she may feel subtly criticised. Third, she may answer from an intellectual position, whereas it would be more helpful to focus on feelings. Fourth, she may not be interested in finding out why; she may rather simply be looking for options to help her cope with her present situation.

Closedness or openness is also conveyed by your tone of voice. It is possible to ask a question that is theoretically closed, such as: 'Do you worry about having cancer?' while at the same time the inflection of your voice invites further disclosure. The patient is then responding more to your sympathetic tone of voice than the words. Similarly, open questions can be asked in a hurried, uninterested way, which may cause the patient to conceal her true feelings.

Either/or questions are variants of closed questions. They aren't usually helpful because there may be more options than are being presented by the questioner, and they can be used to 'lead' the patient.

Leading questions

These are used to persuade, manipulate or coerce the patient into following a course of action that the clinician wants or believes in. An example might be:

Patient: I'm not going to have any more chemotherapy.

Doctor: Don't you think you owe it to your family to have further treatment?'

Again, the verbal message may be backed up by body language that signifies disapproval. As in law courts, leading is inappropriate, but there are subtle variants which are not easily avoided. Some patients want to be led, indeed they expect this of their clinician, and will look for cues as to what they ought to do. They may even put words into their clinician's mouth to justify their decision.

Multiple questions

Radio interviewers like asking politicians several questions at once, and it can be very easy for clinicians to do the same with patients. They may then feel overwhelmed and won't know which to start with and will probably forget the other questions after they have answered one. So, ask one question at a time.

Statements

These can be used as an alternative when questions feel too intrusive. Beginning with such phrases as 'I wonder' or 'I imagine', is a way often used to frame a statement, as with the following:

Question

• What are your concerns about the bone cancer?

Possible related statements

• I wonder what your worries are about having bone cancer.

- I imagine you may have some anxieties about having bone cancer.
- Tell me about your concerns about your bone cancer.

The following transcript highlights the use of reflections, questions and statements.

Althea transcript

Louis: You were saying that you're worried what effect the cancer might have on you.

Althea: Yes. I mean you hear things...

Louis: You hear things?

Althea: Well, my bones could get brittle and even break.

Louis: How do you feel as you tell me this?

Althea: Awful...just awful.

Louis: When you say awful, Althea, what do you mean?

Althea: Well, I just feel so sad and scared...and like I'm falling apart.

Louis: You're falling apart?

Althea: Well, how could I go on if my bones break... I'd... I'd be like one of those rag dolls, just crumpled in a heap.

Louis: A crumpled rag doll...

Althea: Yes...no good for anything... [cries]

Louis: [gently] Althea, what do you imagine that rag doll would need?

Althea: [begins to sob] ... She...she needs to be looked after...

Louis: Yes.

Althea: ... She needs...someone to pick her up and take care of her...

Louis: Is that how you feel, Althea?

Althea: [nods silently; then after a long pause] You know, I had a rag doll like that when I was little... I called her Fin – short for Ragamuffin. I used to carry her with me everywhere... I knew she couldn't take care of herself –

she was so floppy – so I had to look after her…but she
was a wonderful listener. I could tell her anything…

Louis: I wonder who looks after you.

Althea: Oh, I always look after everyone. That's why this illness
is so…frustrating…

Louis: And you?

Althea: [cries] That's what's so hard. I don't like being
dependent on anyone. I need to be in control.

Louis: Otherwise?

Althea: Otherwise it feels terrifying, like a black hole.

This transcript also demonstrates the use of subpersonality and image
work. These will be discussed in the next chapter.

Silence

This is an important counselling skill. We all have an inner psychological
process – the stream of ideas, images and feelings that flows through our
consciousness. These will tend to be linked to one another and reveal
meaningful patterns. Thoughts will always have accompanying feelings,
for example. Freud used this when he asked his patients to free associate, to
tell him their memories, emotions and thoughts as they appeared in
sequence, without censoring them. In this way it was possible to move
beyond their rational defences and discover unconscious psychological
material that related to their presenting complaints. Such thoughts may
appear in profusion or, at times, slow down and even stop. Or a pattern of
ideas appears but needs time to develop. Or a thought may be on the tip of
the tongue. All of these need silence from the listener to avoid disturbing
their gestation; and, at times, silence from the patient for similar reasons.

There are other types of silence – contemplative, embarrassed, angry,
sad, depressed, and so on. One time when it is important to break a silence
is when the patient is losing touch with you. He has withdrawn. Then a
prompt can bring him back in contact with you. A question such as:
'What's happening with you?' may help.

How long is it all right to be silent? As long as necessary. There is no
rule. Marie Cardinal (1993), in her account of her own psychoanalysis,
describes whole sessions where she said nothing. Of course, talking with
patients is different because there is no prearranged agreement to meet for

an hour as there is in counselling. Discussions end when both clinician and patient have finished what they have to say. Nevertheless, silences in the course of such meetings may be appropriate. Some, however, can't tolerate silences of any length and this needs to be respected too.

There is one situation where the contact between clinician and patient may be conducted in total silence: when the latter is dying. If there are no relatives present, this is most often the nurse's territory and the image of the nurse sitting quietly with a patient close to death, holding his hand, is very familiar. I feel this comes within the ambit of counselling skills because it is about being present to the dying person, giving him your attention, just as you would to someone you were talking to. I have not come across many doctors who sit with dying patients, perhaps reflecting the traditional roles that doctors and nurses adopt. Most often, they have experienced this in a personal context, when a relative or friend was dying.

COMBINING CLINICAL AND COUNSELLING SKILLS

In practice, talking with patients will not fall neatly into separate discussions on clinical matters and psychological issues. It is usually a mixture. One of the key skills here is flexibility, the readiness to abandon a prepared list of medical or nursing questions in favour of counselling skills if, for example, emotions surface, and then to return to the clinical history when the patient is ready. The following dialogue gives an example in which elements of breaking bad news appear as well.

Althea transcript

Althea: Well, doctor, I've got to face facts, I know that it's the cancer causing the pain in my spine and I've got to do something about it; I can't sleep at night sometimes and I'm getting cranky with the kids, especially when they jump on me. It really hurts my back.

Louis: And I gather you've tried diclofenac along with codeine, but it's not really controlling the pain. I understand you're going to have some radiotherapy to the painful area next week.

Althea: That's right.

Louis: Well, the next step could be to try a morphine preparation.

Althea: Oh God, I thought you'd say that. I really don't want to take morphine.

Louis: Can you tell me more about that?

Althea: My best friend died of cancer last year and she was put on morphine near the end and...[starts to cry]...she was a complete zombie on it.

Louis: Althea, I imagine it must have been very distressing for you when your friend died. But what about you, what are your concerns?

Althea: Maybe you're telling me I'm going to die soon. [cries]

Louis: To die soon?

Althea: [nods] Yes...and I'm just not ready.

Louis: I can understand that you would feel upset and we can talk further about that in a moment. However, before we go on, it's important to realise that people can be on morphine safely for months or even years. It's given for the pain, and does not imply you are to die soon.

Althea: Oh... I wish I could believe you.

Louis: You're uncertain I'm being honest with you?

Althea: Well...maybe you're just trying to be nice to me.

Louis: What do you think, Althea? We know each other quite well now. Am I someone who would just try to be nice to you?

Althea: [hesitates]... No...you've always been honest with me... I haven't liked it sometimes, but I think I can trust what you say.

In this dialogue, I could, perhaps, have stayed in clinical mode and talked about research evidence or different patients I knew who had been taking morphine for a long time, but by mirroring back to Althea her concerns, she was able to make her own decision, based on her own judgement, that she could trust me.

CHAPTER 5

Psychological Approaches

There are a multitude of schools of counselling and psychotherapy. While a detailed discussion is beyond the scope of this book, there are a number of approaches that are worth considering for the light they throw on working with the dying.

PERSON-CENTRED THERAPY

Carl Rogers (1961, pp.282–4), the founder of humanistic psychology, described six core conditions for constructive personality change to take place in a client, of which three are widely quoted:

1. *Congruence*: this means an accurate matching of experience with awareness by the therapist; in other words that she is fully and accurately aware of what she is experiencing at any moment in her relationship with her client. This has also been described as 'genuineness'. The therapist may share her experience with the client where appropriate. This inner honesty will facilitate trust developing between counsellor and client.

2. *Unconditional positive regard*: Rogers also called this acceptance. He meant the experience of accepting the client's negative as well as positive feelings, of accepting him for who he is and not for what he does, and of respecting his individuality.

3. *Empathy*: this has already been referred to. It means: 'to sense the client's private world as if it were your own, but without ever losing the "as if" quality.'

These important qualities develop over time in a person using counselling skills. It is more a question of uncovering what is already there than of taking on some technical expertise. In all of these, the actual experience of the client and therapist is to the fore, rather than intellectual constructs. It's worth noting that clients usually come to counsellors in a state of incongruence, in other words that their awareness does not match their experience of their body and their feelings. Typical is the client who may say to you angrily: 'I'm not angry'. For therapy to be successful, clients need to have some awareness of the three qualities mentioned above being in their counsellor.

COGNITIVE BEHAVIOURAL THERAPY

Cognitive behavioural therapy (CBT) has become increasingly popular and has been recommended by the National Institute for Clinical Excellence (NICE) as the first-line treatment for depression, based on research evidence for its efficacy in comparison with antidepressants (National Collaborating Centre for Mental Health 2004, pp.129–30). The cognitive aspect (Beck 1989) is based on the observation that every thought has a feeling or feelings linked with it. Furthermore, cognitions may be 'faulty', not in accord with reality. Patients may believe that all people with cancer die in agony or that morphine will kill you (some clinicians think this too). Unsurprisingly, such negative cognitions will be accompanied by distress feelings such as anxiety or depression. Cognitive therapy consists in clarifying what these so-called disordered thoughts are and exploring with the patient their veracity. What is the evidence for their belief? If they can see that their belief is not real, their negative emotions may fade too. It is like the shift in feelings when you realise that the coiled serpent in front of you is actually a coil of rope. Examples of neurotic (as opposed to psychotic) thought disorders include:

- *Personalisation*: the individual overestimates the degrees to which events relate to him.

- *Polarisation*: he thinks in extremes such as always or never. An example is catastrophisation, the assumption that the worst is bound to happen.

- *Arbitrary inference*: he jumps to a conclusion for which evidence is lacking.

Cognitive therapy works with maladaptive thinking. Behavioural therapy works in a similar way with maladaptive behaviour, such as phobias, using graded desensitisation, a process of gradual introduction of the feared object or process. The two approaches overlap and work in the 'here and now', rather than exploring a person's past in search of causes for emotional distress. Thus, in the treatment of bulimia, a potentially life-threatening condition, CBT is used partly to explore the patient's distorted thinking about food, and partly to apply techniques to modify her bingeing and vomiting behaviour.

While CBT requires specialist training, it is still possible to watch for feelings resulting from inaccurate perceptions and investigate these with the patient. It's not surprising that patients with advanced cancer may automatically catastrophise, assuming that *any* new symptom they develop means they are about to die. The evidence for and against such beliefs can be investigated with them. It may not be enough to tell a patient that a symptom is of no serious import. It is at times necessary to find out how they have arrived at their conclusions. Thus, their line of reasoning might be: my uncle died of a brain tumour and had terrible headaches before he died; I have a tumour and I have headaches; so I must have a brain tumour. Once their thought sequence is apparent, it is easier to clarify the logical inconsistencies. The above is an example of arbitrary inference. CBT has been used successfully to treat cancer patients (Moorey and Greer 2002)

A TRANSPERSONAL VIEW

Psychosynthesis, the first transpersonal psychology, was founded by an Italian psychotherapist, Roberto Assagioli (1984). Freud had commented that he was only interested in the basement of human beings. Assagioli responded by saying he was interested in the whole building, including the higher reaches of human nature, its spiritual aspects (Keen 1974, pp.96–104). He sought to redress the Freudian emphasis on sickness by emphasising health in the psyche as well. He developed a map of the psyche as shown in Figure 5.1.

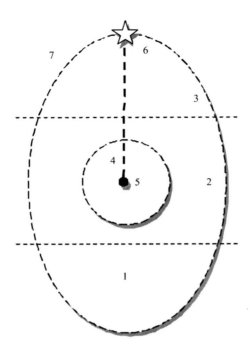

1. The Lower Unconscious
2. The Middle Unconscious
3. The Higher Unconscious or Superconscious
4. The Field of Consciousness
5. The Conscious Self or 'I'
6. The Higher Self
7. The Collective Unconscious

Figure 5.1 Egg diagram (modified from Assagioli 1984, p.14)

Assagioli divided the unconscious into three regions. The lower is that of
our primal instincts. The middle is those elements accessible to our
everyday waking consciousness. The higher is the region of higher intuitions, inspirations, higher feelings, illumination and spiritual energies.
Assagioli felt that these qualities are just as much real aspects of the psyche
as the more well-known elements. While we are familiar with the dark
upwellings of the lower unconscious in the dying, the expression of the

higher unconscious through spiritual experiences also occurs though it may not always be recognised. One woman, for example, described lucidly how she woke one night in a darkened palliative care ward. 'She suddenly experienced lights very brightly, far above her; she looked around but there seemed to be no-one there and everything was silent; this she found extremely beautiful and peaceful and she thought she was dying and in heaven' (Heyse-Moore 1996, p.303). Assagioli also conceptualised the 'I' as being a centre of pure consciousness; this idea will be made use of in meditations described later in this chapter.

SUBPERSONALITIES

Assagioli (Ferrucci 1982, pp.47–58) also described the concept of subpersonalities. We all behave differently in different circumstances of our lives. Thus, I am, by turns, a doctor, husband, father, counsellor, brother and so on. Each of these different roles constellates a set of stable behaviours that changes when we move into another life situation. I remember a striking instance of this when I was a junior doctor. I was in the doctors' mess and a patronising consultant was declaiming his contempt for the poor he dealt with medically. I felt angered by his attitude. The phone rang; it was for him. He listened to the caller and his whole demeanour changed and softened. It was his young children. Gently he told them that Daddy would be home soon. He seemed to have become a different person. My anger turned to amazement at this unlikely transformation.

We all have a wide range of these subpersonalities within us and patients are no exception. Unsurprisingly, there can be trouble. We may be uncomfortable with one of these parts of ourselves, for example an angry aspect. We may be identified with, say, being a victim. Two subpersonalities may clash within us; thus, a part of us that wants to please may be in conflict with another part that wishes to be independent.

Certain subpersonalities are very familiar. Thus we each have an inner Child, whose playfulness and creativity we may value; or we may repress this part as childish and immature. We also each have an inner Critic who, more or less subtly, puts us down: that piece of work was rubbish; you shouldn't waste time gossiping with other staff; you mean you don't know about that? And so on. This character represents an internalisation of the throng of shoulds and shouldn'ts we have all absorbed from our parents, school, university and place of work. Another is the Victim, overwhelmed and helpless in the face of bad fortune; he is oppressed by the Bully who lives up to his name. Note that both of these subpersonalities can coexist as polarities in the same person.

Dying patients can exhibit a wide variety of subpersonalities. The Victim is a common one. Another is the Fighter, who, against insuperable odds is determined to beat the cancer, St George slaying the dragon. The Blue Peter presenter, Caron Keating, spent over £1 million travelling the world, seeking out a multitude of complementary therapies, before she died of disseminated breast cancer. A frequent and sad scenario is the patient who desperately insists that his oncologist gives him further chemotherapy which they both know has little or no chance of helping and may actually make him worse. Then there is the Joker, who laughs to stop himself crying. Or the Rationaliser who tries to understand his illness intellectually, but ignores his feelings. Or the person who scurries around like a worker ant trying to keep himself busy because otherwise he would have to let in his emptiness and inner pain - this is the so called manic defence.

Subpersonalities can be a useful way of viewing patient behaviour and working with it:

- The simplest method of doing this is in terms of awareness of what is happening. Thus: 'So, it seems like there's a victim part of you that feels helpless and there's another part of you that is determined to fight the cancer.'

- Another way is to ask the patient to describe an image that comes to him of a particular subpersonality. Thus, one woman described a grieving part of herself as dull, tattered, old and depressed. This makes the experience more vivid. It is then possible to converse, as it were, with this image internally. Suitable questions might be: 'If this image could speak, what would she be saying to you?' or 'What would you like to say to this part of you?' In this way, a dialogue can be established and an ignored subpersonality is given space to speak, to communicate its message which may well be pertinent, if unwelcome, to the patient.

- This is a powerful way of working because it functions at the imaginal level and thus bypasses the mental censorship that so often inhibits awareness of our psychological processes – the part of us that says: 'That's silly' or: 'It's wrong to be angry' and so on.

- Remember, a disliked subpersonality may actually be serving a useful purpose. Thus some people become compulsive carers as a way of appeasing their chronic sense of guilt instilled by condemning parents. Others become melancholic as a way of blanking out unbearable inner distress, like a fog. While this is obviously not ideal, it was the method that they developed, perhaps in childhood, of surviving. It may have outlived its purpose, indeed it may be destructive now, but it is important not to force a patient to change, to destabilise her coping mechanisms, before she is ready. Subpersonality work allows her to explore the roots of her inner conflicts, her times of feeling stuck, gradually so that change can take place organically when she is ready.

Visualisation will be discussed in more detail later in this chapter.

ARCHETYPES

Carl Jung (Storr 1998, pp.65–85) proposed the existence of a collective unconscious, common to all humanity of which each individual unconscious is an aspect. He also described archetypes. These are the foundation stones of the collective unconscious and so of our individual psyches, the stuff of which our inner worlds are made. We encounter images of these archetypes in mythologies, fairy tales, poetry, music and the sacred books of many religions. Their presence is felt as awe-inspiring and powerful.

Archetypes make themselves known compellingly in palliative care. The most obvious is Death, often imagined as the skeletal Grim Reaper, dressed in a hooded black cloak. The sense of terror and awe evoked by this image was used effectively by Charles Dickens in his book, *A Christmas Carol*, in which Scrooge meets the spectral Ghost of Christmas Future, a fearful prophet of the miser's lonely demise. For cancer patients, the Crab can be a symbol of the deadly, spreading potential of their disease. Curiously, another image, death as the Kindly Angel, is not often evoked, though many patients will see death as a welcome release. We need to be aware that the archetype of mortality is present to every dying patient – and, for that matter, to staff as well. Some deny, some are terrified, some accept, but all are affected. Much of the work around the anxiety or despair that dying people feel is, whether stated or not, about the fear of Death, and what he portends.

Another important archetype is of Healing. This has already been considered in Chapter 1 where we saw that it is not only about physical cure but about a state of wholeness and relatedness, even when dying. Patients will project this quality onto staff, particularly doctors and nurses. While clinicians do function in a healing capacity, much work with the dying is to help them to find their own inner healing – of their psyche and their spirit. It is seductive, yet untrue, to imagine that we clinicians are the bringers of all healing. In truth, there have been many patients in whose presence I have felt healed, just as much as the other way round. This speaks to a like archetype, the Wounded Healer, exemplified by the myth of Chiron the centaur who searched for years for a cure for his deadly, incurable wound; his discoveries made him a great healer to whom sick people flocked (Kearney 1996). Each one of us, whether clinician or patient, carries this psychological configuration.

The Mother is another significant archetype in hospice care. Many patients have had difficult childhoods, experiencing conflict, loneliness and a lack of love. It is common in palliative care to see very frail bed-bound patients being fed, washed and turned by the nurses. While this may be necessary physically, it may also be the first time in decades that they have experienced real care, given with the love that a mother gives to her child. I remember how Jean Vanier, founder of L'Arche, communities for people with learning difficulties, described a visit to an institute for the long-term care of children with severe disabilities in France. It was a grim place. Some inmates were chained to the wall. He came across a boy who lived in a cot with bars; his mother could not bear to come and visit him. Jean picked the boy up and he felt him trembling with delight at the physical contact of which he had so long been starved. (Note how men can give mothering too.) In fact, a major part of the ambience of hospices is about providing a secure place which holds and contains the distress experienced by the dying.

The Hero is another prevalent archetype. This is a major part of acute medicine with its emphasis on battling with death – both the patient and staff participate in this form of heroism. Palliative care does not overtly subscribe to this philosophy and yet the wish to stave off death just a little longer can still persist. One more course of antibiotics for pneumonia;

another blood transfusion. It would seem these are for symptom control purposes, but maybe we also try them sometimes at the patient's behest even when we know they are unlikely to work. Doctors are particularly prone to assume the heroic mantle – it is so flattering! – and one of the changes of attitude that doctors new to hospice work painfully have to learn is the letting go of their familiar heroic technology of cure. It has been a familiar sight for me to see new doctors on the hospice ward struggling with the prospect of *not* doing investigations and acute therapies.

A different form of heroic myth in palliative care is that every suffering the patient experiences can be quickly relieved – whether of pain, depression or isolation. While it's true that physical symptoms can be treated, often with spectacular success, psychologically it is not so simple. There may not be enough time to address in depth a patient's long-term depression or anxiety; their family conflicts may be deep-seated. Counselling skills need time to be effective in these situations. If a person only has a week or so to live and doesn't wish to talk, it may be that tranquillisers are the only measure that will help to relieve his psychic pain. And to make matters worse, he may even refuse these. Let's be aware, then, of the limits of our heroism. Sometimes, what is most helpful is simply to sit with a person when he is dying – 'Watch with me' was one of Dame Cicely Saunders' favourite sayings.

Archetypal images can be worked with in the same way as indicated for subpersonalities. In fact the latter may have archetypal qualities to them – the Warrior is an example.

MEDITATION AND VISUALISATION

Meditation is associated with the following physiological changes (LeShan 1999, pp.42–6):

- reduced respiratory and heart rate, and blood pressure
- lowered metabolic rate
- reduced blood lactate concentration (anxiety causes high concentrations)
- increased skin resistance (low resistance occurs with anxiety)
- brain wave changes, typically an increase in slow alpha waves.

These changes – the so-called relaxation response (Benson 1996) – do not occur during hypnosis or sleep. They are the reverse of the stress response and so have many potential benefits in palliative care:

- to reduce psychological distress such as anxiety, panic attacks or agitation

- as a way of working on the patient's psychological process

- as self-care exercises that staff can use for themselves.

Examples of meditations are given here. Spiritual aspects of meditation are discussed in Chapter 10.

For all the following exercises, ask the patient to get in a comfortable position, preferably sitting up with a straight back since this helps concentration and eases breathing if there are respiratory problems. Some patients, however, because of their frailty or paralysis, for example, may need to be lying down. The instructions are written here as you would say them to the patient. Speak slowly and quietly and pause to allow silence between each statement so that the patient has time to experience what you have said in his body.

Meditation – muscle relaxation

- Close you eyes or, if you prefer, keep them half open and look softly at a spot a few feet in front of you.

- Become aware of your breathing... Notice your in-breath and your out-breath...there is no need to change anything, just become aware... Notice the sensation of the air flowing in and out of your nostrils.

- Now become aware of your feet... Notice any sensations in them... There is no need to change anything, just notice the sensations... Now let your feet relax and the muscles soften and loosen... If it helps, imagine that there have been rubber bands wound round your feet and these are now unwinding... Feel your feet supported by the bed (or floor, or cushion)...let in the security and solidity of that support.

- Now move your awareness to your legs.

- (The same sequence of instructions is repeated for the legs.)

- (This is then repeated for the pelvis, the back, the stomach, the chest [here ask them to focus on the chest moving as they

breathe], the arms, the neck and the head. If indicated, the
exercise can be done in more detail, for example the lower back
or the face. This might apply if there are symptoms affecting a
particular part of the body.)

- Now become aware of your breathing again... No need to
  change anything.

- When you are ready, come back into the room and open your
  eyes.

Don't rush this meditation. It may take 15–20 minutes to go through the
entire sequence. Allow the patient time to reconnect with you afterwards.
It's useful to ask him what his experience was. Almost always patients find
this exercise very calming. They may find that breathlessness and pain are
reduced. It is not, however, a magic bullet that solves all problems in one
go. It is important to do this meditation regularly daily, and at other times
when required, for example if they feel a panic attack coming on. Give the
patient a printed sheet of instructions so that he can remember them. For
those whose concentration is impaired by their illness or their medications,
staff or family can repeat the instructions to them, or they can be recorded
on a tape. Similar commercial relaxation tapes or CDs are available on the
internet. Even patients who seem quite sleepy may be able to use this
meditation.

It might be argued that focusing on a painful area could worsen the
pain. In practice, the opposite is usually true. The conscious act of noticing
a symptom such as pain causes a degree of mental separation from it, so
that patients are no longer lost in an agitated identification with their
distress. As their anxiety lessens, this leads to an actual reduction of their
pain. A benign, rather than vicious, circle is set in motion. I have also found
that, if I do this exercise with a patient, I usually feel calmer myself at the
end – a useful spin-off for busy clinicians.

I remember one elderly woman dying of lung cancer who was very
breathless and anxious. I did the above meditation with her and watched
with fascination as her anxiety, tension and breathlessness melted away.
She seemed to be particularly in tune with this approach and she died
comfortably three days later without even having to repeat the exercise.

Meditation – pure consciousness

- Close you eyes or, if you prefer, keep them half open and focus softly on a spot a few feet in front of you.

- Become aware of your breathing… Notice your in-breath and your out-breath…there is no need to change anything, just become aware… Notice the sensation of the air flowing in and out of your nostrils.

- Notice that there is an aspect of you that is conscious of your breathing, a centre of awareness observing your respirations.

- Stay with that awareness. Keep returning to it every time your mind wanders, using your breathing to help you do this.

This meditation relates to the principle of disidentification, as discussed by Assagioli (1984, pp.213–17). So often, we become identified with symptoms such as chronic pain or anxiety so that these states seem to fill the whole of our consciousness. Simply noticing the suffering can be used as a way of gaining some psychological space, a recognition that your awareness is *more than* your emotional or physical distress:

Meditation – mindfulness of pain

- Start as for the previous meditation by becoming aware of your breathing.

- Slowly scan your body. Imagine that, as you breathe, the breath flows into and out of the area you are focusing on.

- Be aware of any areas of pain.

- Don't try to change them, simply be aware of them.

- Try to observe the pain as an immediate felt experience – How would you describe it? What is its quality? Where is it in your body? Does it wax and wane? And so on.

- If you feel any emotions such as fear, again simply notice them as for the pain.

- Once you have spent some time with one area of pain, move on to the next part of your body, then return to your breathing at the end.

Does this steady awareness of the pain aggravate it? The opposite is true as has been demonstrated by Kabat-Zinn (1990) who has used this approach, which he calls the practice of mindfulness, successfully in relieving chronic pain, both malignant and non-malignant. It is not, however, a quick fix. It usually takes time and persistence to gain benefit from this and so is more helpful for those who still have some time left to live.

Visualisation has been used by a variety of psychological schools. Jung, for example, developed 'active imagination' as a way of having a dialogue with the unconscious (Johnson 1986).

Visualisation – a lake in the country – first part

- Close you eyes or, if you prefer, keep them half open and focus softly on a spot a few feet in front of you.

- Become aware of your breathing... Notice your in-breath and your out-breath...there is no need to change anything, just become aware... Notice the sensation of the air flowing in and out of your nostrils.

- Imagine that you are sitting near a lake in the country. It could be one you have actually visited or it might be one you make up in your imagination.

- Look around this peaceful place and notice what you see...perhaps there are trees and bushes...flowers...maybe there is grass surrounding the lake... The sun is shining and you can see clouds drifting across the blue sky... Are there any birds?... Look at the lake sparkling blue in the sunshine... Maybe there are reeds in a shallow part of the lake... What else can you see?

- What can you hear?... Perhaps the wind blowing in the trees... The sounds of birds calling... The lapping of water at the edge of the lake.

- Notice your body sensations where you are sitting... Be aware of what you are sitting on, perhaps grass... Maybe your back is resting against a tree... If so, feel the roughness of the bark...sense the wind blowing, its coolness on your skin... Touch the ground with your hand... What do you feel?

- What scents or smells are there?... Flowers?... The clean smell of water from the lake?... The scent of pine?... Anything else?

- Take your time and enjoy being in this peaceful place. Walk around for a while if you wish.

- Take your leave of the lake and return to this room. Remember you can always return to this place whenever you like.

This visualisation is particularly powerful because it involves images from the subject's memory that he associates with calmness, enjoyment and relaxation. Note that 'image' here relates to any and all of the senses, each of which is evoked in turn and this heightens the feeling of reality, of being in the scene itself. There are many variations of this type of visualisation, depending on what the subject finds works best for her. She might, for example, choose a different scene such as a mountain valley, or a beach. There is no need to use the suggested examples above. If she is by the sea, she may choose to recall the smell of salt in the air and the sound of waves breaking. There are many CDs available of natural sounds, panpipe music and so on that some people find helpful as a background while they meditate.

This approach can, too, be developed further. For example, the meditation can be extended to facilitate contact with the higher unconscious as a source of inner advice and wisdom. The exercise follows the same pattern as already described in the first part of the visualisation. Before coming out of it, the following is added:

Visualisation – a lake in the country – second part

- Down by the lake you can see a person in the far distance. You know that this person is wise, cares deeply for you and your welfare, and has a message for you... He or she is walking slowly towards you...

- I invite you, if you wish, to go down to the lake and meet this person...

- As you approach, see who this person is...

- Greet him or her in whatever way feels appropriate to you...

- Listen to the message...

- See if there is any response you wish to make...

- Take your leave of this person and then of the lake...

- When you are ready, come back into the room and open your eyes.

This seemingly simple exercise can have a very intense and emotive effect. One woman described how she met her dead grandmother, whose message was very simply that she would be all right. The woman found this inner encounter profoundly reassuring and supportive. She didn't imagine that she would suddenly be cured of her cancer, rather that she would be looked after, and her feelings of distress reduced markedly. How could such an obvious statement be so helpful? Maybe it is because this exercise works at the archetypal level where profound significance attaches to any words used. We all experience this when listening to a beautiful and haunting song – the tune adds depth and meaning to the lyrics which might sound quite banal if just spoken.

Visualisations can be used in other ways, though these require training for their effective implementation:

- to converse with a subpersonality or archetypal image
- to imagine a dialogue between two subpersonalities
- imagining speaking with a real person to resolve interpersonal issues.

The recommended reading list at the end of this book gives details of books which explore this further.

WORKING WITH DREAMS

To work with dreams is to step into a vast unconscious world whose laws are profoundly different from our external reality. As with all of us, dying people dream and may be disturbed by their dreams. There are some simple guidelines that can be used to help them find meaning in their dreams.

First, the language of dreams is that of metaphors and symbols. They are like poetry, mythology or fairy tales in this respect. Therefore, trying to ascribe a literal meaning to dreams won't work. In particular, dreams about death may not necessarily be about death at all. The psyche may simply be using death as a metaphor for transitions. This is obviously important if a patient with advanced cancer has such a dream. He may think it means he is about to die, whereas exploration of the dream may reveal an altogether different interpretation.

Second, events in dreams have an individual significance for each individual. A dream about flying may have different meanings for different people. Dream manuals that assign set connotations for themes such as journeys, animals, loss of an object and so on, shut the door to discovering the unique significance of a dream for a particular person. Having said this, one way of looking at dreams is to hypothesise that each figure represents some aspect of the dreamer and his life, even though they may apparently be their father or daughter or friend and so on. Inanimate objects such as a house can equally represent the dreamer. Dreams may be seen as the psyche commenting on a person's life and they may be compensatory – that is they address the very thing that in waking life the dreamer represses. They are, then, a method of psychological self-regulation. No wonder we sometimes have nightmares – they may be trumpet calls from the unconscious waking us from our conscious denial.

Many people dismiss dreams as foolish and ignore them because they do not follow the physical and biological laws of our everyday lives. However, we do not dismiss a painting by Giotto of angels, or Dante's *The Divine Comedy* or Mozart's opera *The Magic Flute* simply because they involve fantasy – indeed the material for these works of art must have come from their authors' unconscious. Why not treat dreams as seriously as you would such creations?

Here are some ways of approaching a patient's dream (Johnson 1986):

- Does he want to work on the dream? If not, respect this, however intriguing it may be.

- Ask him to tell you the story of the dream.

- What are his initial impressions?

- How does each figure relate to the others? What is each figure wanting?

- Ask him to free associate around figures in the dream. This means allowing any thoughts, images, feelings or sensations to appear without censorship, even if they seem strange, that he associates with each figure. Often, one particular association will 'click' as fitting best.

- Beware of pronouncing your own interpretations, however brilliant they may seem. Your job is to help the dreamer find his own meaning.

- Give it time. It may take several days or longer before it becomes clear what the dream is saying.

Kearney (1996, pp.129–34) recounts a remarkable dream told to him by a patient, James, who was dying of advanced oesophageal cancer. He was pale, ill, frightened and breathless. In his dream, he was led to Newgrange, a prehistoric burial chamber in Ireland. 'He led him into the heart of the tomb, so that James's back rested on the stone slab which is touched by the first rays of sun each midwinter's day.' He was then led out of the burial chamber and instructed to dig. He found a marvellous 'pre-ancient city' and could see the outlines of the houses and the streets. After this dream, he was transformed. He lost his fears and his symptoms abated. He died peacefully two weeks later. Outwardly, his situation was no different, but inwardly his perception of the meaning of his life and death had undergone a radical change; a true healing.

THE PRESENTING PAST

It is such a cliché: I want to put the past behind me. The truth, however, is often otherwise. Unhealed, painful memories are repressed and relegated into the shadows of the unconscious, but they do not tamely stay hidden. They make their presence felt in unaccountable changes of mood – depression or anxiety for example – or in our emotional reactions to people we meet who remind us of someone from our past. To our surprise, anger or coldness, say, suffuse such meetings. We do not want it so, but it happens.

Psychodynamic counselling (Jacobs 1998) explores the past of an individual, searching for the origins of his presenting distress: childhood abuse, family conflicts, bullying at school and so on. Developmental psychology (Winnicott 1988) focuses on what the normal development of a person is and where this may have gone astray. An example would be of a daughter who gives up her teenage years to take care of her single, disabled mother, who is slowly dying of multiple sclerosis. The daughter, then, misses out on the experience of adolescence necessary for her psychological transition to adulthood.

While these are specialist types of therapy, any clinician can still be mindful of a person's past and listen for clues connecting his past life with his present distress. One of the hardest things I had to do when I was a house physician was to tell a twelve-year-old boy, whose mother had died a year or so before, that his father, who had just been admitted to hospital, had suddenly died too. I can still remember his frozen, wide-eyed face as I talked to him. I can only imagine the effect it must have had on him and how it marked him for life. Although I spoke to him as gently as I could, I had no skills in supporting a teenager in such a tragedy nor in knowing who could help him. Left unresolved, such traumas may resurface when another stressful life event triggers them off. Perhaps more than anything else, dying will re-evoke the past.

Doctors, nurses and social workers working with the dying will all take some kind of family history. This usually acts as a catalyst for revealing past life issues. Similarly, a simple enquiry about whether the patient has had any difficult times in his life can be used in this context. Hints may be dropped by the patient and these can be followed up. One man told me that his young daughter had died in a car accident some 40 years before but he had put it behind him; he firmly told me he didn't want to talk about it. While it was important to respect his wish, over time it became apparent that he hadn't got over his daughter's death – it was a significant aspect of his chronic psychological distress.

TEAM COUNSELLING SUPPORT

Counselling skills are most often used to provide support for a patient who is already troubled. Some patients are admitted to a hospice apparently coping. Then they talk to the staff for the first time about the prospect of dying. Memories of past unresolved traumas surface. Suddenly they are plunged into crisis, requiring intensive multidisciplinary team support. This will obviously be sustaining, but at the same time, it is a big advantage if one of those involved is a trained counsellor with the psychological skills to support such a patient. Often, it is the social worker who plays this role and who can help coordinate the support other members of the team provide.

Part 2
Palliative Care Issues

CHAPTER 6

Breaking Bad News

THE NECESSITY OF BREAKING BAD NEWS

In Ancient Greece, the envoy bringing bad tidings was killed, presumably to ward off the bad luck he brought. Why, I sometimes wonder, would anyone in those times wish to be such a messenger? Nowadays, bearers of bad news are not treated so drastically, but they still aren't welcomed. It's no wonder, then, if we go back a mere 50 years, that doctors, for it was always doctors then, did not usually tell patients if they had cancer. The doctors lied, used euphemisms such as 'inflammation' or avoided the question altogether. They wanted to avoid causing pain. It was considered good practice, however, to tell the family, and this set up a barrier of silence between the ill person and her loved ones.

The situation now is very different, much of this due to the work of the Hospice Movement in this area. It is so different that guidelines from the General Medical Council (2006, p.16) to doctors insist that it is an ethical duty to tell patients what is wrong with them. Furthermore, such information can only be given to the family with the patients' consent. A revolution indeed, and a good one.

Of course breaking bad news will cause distress; there is no getting round that. But there is a deeper imperative. Each individual has a right to be respected. He has a right to know about his illness. To deny him this is to infantilise him. How else can he decide what action to take – what treatment to have, what to say to his family?

Are there ever occasions, then, when one should not break bad news to an ill person? These are few, but include the following:

- the person who makes it clear he does not want to be told

- the demented person whose loss of memory means she has forgotten what you told her half an hour later. Repeating the information means she undergoes the same emotional reaction repeatedly – a needless cruelty
- the confused patient who cannot take in the information
- psychotic patients who are liable to incorporate the information you give them into their paranoid delusions.

THE PARTICIPANTS

Apart from the patient himself, family members are often in attendance when the bad news is being given and may take part in the subsequent discussion. If there are many relatives present, this may detract from the time which needs to be given to the ill person. The information provided will not only affect each person present individually but also how they relate to each other in the meeting; hidden conflicts may be revealed. I can remember sitting at the bedside of a patient with advanced cancer and being asked by him if he was dying. This was a moment of opportunity that I felt could not be missed; he had avoided asking about his illness before. But, out of sight behind him, his wife was frantically waving her arms at me to stop me from answering. I was in a dilemma, but felt I had to proceed – he had the right to an honest answer from his doctor and it was, after all, his illness – and I told him he was indeed dying. After this I asked his wife if she wanted to say anything, but she declined. It left me with a bad taste in my mouth. Perhaps, with hindsight, it might have been better to bring her silent attempt at prohibition into the conversation; but I knew, too, that the patient would then have changed the subject; he never overtly opposed his wife. Giving him the news about his condition also high-lighted the fact that his wife had withheld this from him, fertile territory for anger on his part and guilt on hers.

Another scenario I encountered frequently took place on home visits. I would be welcomed into the house and steered into the sitting room, although the patient was upstairs in his bedroom. A group of family members would then inform me that the patient had not been told that he was dying or even, sometimes, that he had cancer and they were concerned to ensure that I wouldn't upset him by telling him. Finding an answer that maintained communication was awkward. I usually said I certainly wouldn't give him any information that he didn't want, but if he did ask about his illness then he had a right to know. This was almost always enough for the family and we could then proceed to see the patient. What amazed me was how often patients *did* then ask about their illness in the presence of their partner. They would say they knew they were dying and we had the surreal situation that both partners were trying to protect each other from knowledge that they both already knew. When they realised this, the relief was almost palpable; it was as though an invisible wall between them had been removed. These were often very moving moments, points of healing in their relationship which had been put under strain by the barrier of silence between them.

The person breaking the bad news needs to understand enough about the patient's illness and treatment to be able to answer her or her family's questions. In the past this was the province of the doctor, but nowadays nurses trained in palliative care also take on this role. This particularly applies for community nurse specialists who work alone visiting patients at home; often they are the ones who talk most with these patients about their condition. Social workers and counsellors can then capitalise on the patient's insight and explore her feelings further. Ministers, similarly, can address the spiritual questions patients may have about their impending death. It is often useful for more than one discipline to work together in breaking bad news. Most often, this will be the doctor and nurse, but the social worker may be involved too.

Finally, family members themselves may decide to give this information, with or without the presence of a staff member. This sharing can enhance the intimacy between them and the patient. It is important, however, to check later the understanding gained in this process. Information given may be factually incorrect or, perhaps, certain parts might be withheld as too distressing to talk about. There are cultural issues to be considered, too. These will be addressed in more detail in Chapter 9.

THE PLACE

In palliative care units, a room where conversations can take place privately is obviously best but, unfortunately, not always attainable, as previously discussed. The exception is breaking bad news to family separately from the patient since they are usually able to walk to a private room. It is preferable that those involved are sitting. Apart from the implied sense of equality this imparts, from a pragmatic point of view if one of those present is standing and feels faint or shocked at the news, he might fall and injure himself.

THE BAD NEWS

This usually concerns one of the following:

- the diagnosis of cancer or another life-threatening illness
- the treatment and its consequences:
  - toxicity of chemotherapy
  - loss of a body part such as limb amputation
  - mutilation
- the failure of treatment
- no treatment is possible
- the illness is progressing
- loss of function such as paralysis
- dying
- the sudden death or serious illness of someone close to the patient.

Breaking bad news, then, is not a once and for all task. It is a process that keeps pace with each new circumstance of the patient's illness.

With the shift in culture around breaking bad news, most patients have already been told their diagnosis by the time they are referred to a palliative care service. A new problem has resulted. The pendulum may swing the other way. Some patients have told me how they were informed about their diagnosis brusquely and insensitively. They were given too much information too fast, with little regard for their feelings. While most clinicians will handle this issue with care, some do not find it easy and overcompensate, forcing themselves to say what they shy away from and so coming across as uncaring. This may partly be an effect of the ongoing radical transition in clinical practice towards sharing information with patients but it has to be said that some clinicians have a better feel for this than others.

CHECKING IN

Before launching into telling a patient or her family the bad news, it may be helpful to spend a few minutes chatting, finding out how she has been getting on. If she knows that the interview is about her illness and treatment, she will inevitably be anxious. The very act of talking helps to reduce the tension she will be feeling and she may well tell you immediately what her main concerns are.

SIGNALLING

The next step is to give her a warning signal as to the purpose of the meeting. For example: 'So, we're here today to talk about the results of your tests.' You can then ask, if she hasn't already told you, whether she has any particular questions or worries that she would like addressed. It is important to remember these and to return to them at the appropriate moment.

GIVING THE BAD NEWS

There are a number of points to bear in mind:

Keep it simple

It is all too easy, particularly for doctors, to get lost in a welter of jargon. Try to imagine what it is like for the person you talk to, what her level of understanding is. It's better to err on the side of oversimplification; the patient or her family can then ask for more detail if they wish. If you tell her that she has a widespread renal carcinoma with multiple bony metastases, she probably won't understand renal or carcinoma or metastases. Instead talk about a kidney cancer that has spread to the bones.

Go slowly

This is hard for busy clinicians, but essential. You need to slow down almost to one fact at a time. Start, for example, with: 'You have a cancer.' ...pause... 'A cancer of the kidney.' ...pause... 'The cancer has spread to your bones.' ...pause... 'The bones of your spine.'

Stop frequently

Although I have simply put in pauses above, keep looking at her and gauging her reaction. It may be that the first fact is as much as she can take in. Therefore, be prepared to stop until she is ready to go on. One man, when given the diagnosis of cancer described the sense of shock, as if he'd been struck in the pit of his stomach, when he heard the word cancer. He felt a mixture of freezing and of panic so that he was hardly able to hear what the doctor was saying next.

Repetition

Because of the sense of shock, it may be necessary to repeat information many times before it sinks in. I remember one woman kept returning to this as we talked. 'So, you think it's cancer, then, doctor?' she said; then a few minutes later: 'It's cancer, is it?' She repeated this several times in the course of the interview, while I gently confirmed she was right every time she asked. It was as much as she could absorb.

Use neutral language

Avoid making value judgements about the bad news. Thus: 'The operation showed that you have a cancer of the breast which also affects your armpit', rather than: 'I'm sorry to tell you that you have a really nasty breast cancer that has spread to your armpit which is bad news I'm afraid.' The second version sets the patient up to go into a hopeless, victim state. She already has enough to contend with as she deals with her own feelings about discovering she has cancer.

Some doctors in acute medical specialties tell their patients they have either a male or a female cancer. I presume they are referring to its speed of growth. Personally, I don't like this description. Quite apart from the sexist assumption that men are active and women passive, it doesn't do justice to the huge variation in how quickly cancers grow. Isn't it simpler to say that this cancer is slow-growing, or that another usually tends to grow quickly, but that this varies with individuals?

Another phraseology I don't like is the opening gambit: 'I have good news and bad news'. Once more, it sets up expectations in the patient. She may not think the good news is good news. She may actually want to die soon because she wants to be with her dead husband. Just let it be news and then deal with the patient's reactions.

Remember, too, to check with the patient what her understanding of cancer is. You may get some surprises. One man told me that he had been informed at various times that he had a tumour, a growth and a malignancy. He thought these were all different illnesses.

Be honest

Apart from the ethical imperative, patients and their families can often tell if you're lying to them. This immediately sets up a barrier of mistrust between you, of which you are part, since you know you have been dishonest. This does not mean that you have to give patients every available crumb of information on the cancer or the side-effects of the chemotherapy, complete with the latest research findings. Some patients will want that and they will soon be busy trawling the internet and scouring drug data sheets to check up on what you have said. Most just want to know the main headings of how it will affect them or to speak of fears they may have of some complication. They will want to rely on your judgement as an expert, but they need to know that they can ask freely about anything that concerns them. Be prepared, too, to say: 'I don't know'. Often, there are no clear answers as to what exactly will happen with the cancer or its treatment.

Emotions

Just about any emotion can appear during this process. Perhaps the most common are shock and tearfulness. Patients may say that it seems unreal. This is a defence mechanism – dissociation – which numbs the painfulness of what they are hearing. Their feelings may then come through hours, days or even occasionally weeks later. They may feel fear: 'I'm afraid of dying.' Anger is often displaced: 'I'm going to complain about my GP who missed the diagnosis', but may also appear as a rage against their illness: 'Just cut the damned thing out.' There may be shame at having such a 'defiling' illness or guilt at not being able to be the breadwinner any more. Denial is another unconscious strategy. I recall one man who was admitted to a hospice where I was working. He had been working closely with an adviser in the field of alternative therapies who had convinced him that he didn't have cancer at all; if he believed strongly enough that it was an illusion, then it wouldn't exist. He ignored tests that clearly demonstrated his cancer, nor did he acknowledge the obvious mass in his abdomen.

While it would be easy simply to to blame his adviser, the patient himself must have found this strategy preferable at an unconscious level to letting in the pain of his diagnosis.

There needs to be a balance, then, between the active process of information-giving and the receptive process of support during the ensuing emotional reactions.

Treatment decisions

Hand in hand with news about the diagnosis go questions about treatment. By definition, palliative care patients will not be curable but there are a wide range of therapies that provide remission or palliation. For cancer patients, this will usually involve radiotherapy, chemotherapy or surgery. While they will be advised by their surgeon or oncologist, patients will often discuss these options as part of their palliative care, and this is most likely to be with a doctor because of the level of technical knowledge needed. What I find striking is how often they are prepared to try almost anything in the hope of keeping the cancer at bay. They will accept, for example, the high toxicity of chemotherapies, even those that have a low remission rate or are experimental. Their will to survive is remarkable. I recall one woman with breast cancer who had a phobia of needles and of being injected with toxic drugs. Yet she felt she had to keep going for the sake of her family. So she endured the treatments and the attendant panic attacks. I could only watch and admire her resolution.

This, equally, is a difficult problem for oncologists. How are they to decide on the balance between worthwhile levels of remission rates and toxicity of treatment? And if a patient is desperately pleading for one more course of chemotherapy, what should they say in doubtful cases?

Making sure the patient has a clear understanding of what the treatment involves, its likely side-effects and outcome, facilitates discussing what their hopes are for the course of their illness. They may be very unrealistic, imagining that that they will have another 10 or 15 years of life when, actually, the chemotherapy may only buy them another few months at most.

Other patients, however, are undecided. This particularly applies for older patients who are used to being told what to do by their doctors. It is hard for them to take on the responsibility of choosing. They may ask you what you would do. It is important to avoid going down this road. You are an individual, different from them, and what is right for you may not be right for them. It is better to explore their feelings for and against further treatment, their hopes, their anxieties, and give them time to reflect. They may wish to go away and talk with their family, then return in a few days with their decision.

Another reason for patients making their own decisions is that it helps them to re-empower themselves in a situation where they often feel helpless and at the mercy of their illness. Similarly, while not avoiding the bad news, part of the interview can be used to focus on what actions, in addition to the above acute medical treatment decisions, *can* be taken, and this may be almost anything: medications to relieve pain; a stay in the hospice to give their partner a rest; researching on the internet; talking with their children; involving their minister if they so wish; planning a last holiday; and so on. Patients may not feel ready to talk about all such issues in one interview, but they can be followed up at later meetings. The message is: they are still alive; they still have strengths.

If a patient is not able to make a decision himself because, for example, of confusion or dementia, then it is important to talk with the family and the rest of the multidisciplinary team to assess what the patient would have wanted. Almost always a consensus is achieved. Families do not, however, have the ultimate right to decide on a patient's further treatment, even if they think they do. In the rare cases where there is disagreement, it is important for the doctor, who has in such situations to make the final medical decision, to explain the patient's reasoning to the family and to talk through their concerns with them. If patients are so ill they are unable to decide on their treatment, it is unlikely they will be suitable for taxing oncological therapies. It is more likely that discussion with the family will centre around palliative treatments such as antibiotics for pneumonia, blood transfusions or glucocorticosteroids for brain metastases.

Prognosis

Patients and relatives almost always ask: 'How long have I got?' Here, the saying that there are lies, damned lies and statistics has some truth in it. For a start, no two patients are identical even if they are at a similar stage in their illness. Each will react individually to their illness. Some research suggests, for example, that those determined to fight may survive longer than those who despair and give up (LeShan 1994) though this has been disputed by other studies. Second, prognosis estimates depend on accurate staging and patients referred to hospices may not have been staged recently. Third, even if prognostic data are available for a particular stage of a particular cancer, this is only an average. Imagine this were, for the sake of argument, six months. Actually, this means that for a group of cancer patients at the same stage there will be a range of survival between a few weeks and several years, with a mean of six months. To tell a patient she has a prognosis of six months in this case will almost certainly be wrong. You have no way of knowing where on the survival range she will fall. You might get some idea by observing how fast the cancer is progressing, but this is not an exact science. Many studies have shown doctors to be poor estimators of prognosis (Heyse-Moore and Johnson-Bell 1987) perhaps because they so infrequently see the natural course of an illness unaffected by treatment.

It doesn't help a patient and his family to be told a figure and then to find that he is still alive on the dreaded date that they have all been anticipating with such fear. I have talked to many dying people in this situation and they are often, understandably, angry. Better, then, to say that you don't know, or, if you do use statistics, make very sure they understand there is a wide spread of survival for cancer patients at their particular stage. Sometimes, a fuzzy wording such as 'weeks to months' or 'days to weeks' can be used. This is a possible compromise as long as you feel sure of your ground and qualify what you say with a comment on ranges. The very act of estimating the prognosis to be under a year may still come as a shock to those terminally ill patients who still imagine they have ten years to live. Of course they may go into denial anyway and still believe they have that length of time. Conversely, some patients who are clearly close to death fear that their life will drag on painfully for months on end. They may be relieved to know they have *not* got long to live. However, it is obviously important to find out their feelings about dying *before* imparting this information.

A frequent question in respect of cancer patients who are close to death, is: should relatives living overseas or on holiday be called yet? My answer is almost always yes, simply because there is no room for error. If an overseas family member puts off his flight, he may arrive after the patient has died. It is better to arrive early – if that is a suitable term in such circumstances – to ensure that goodbyes can be said.

Ending the interview

Those taking part may need time after the meeting to sit quietly for a while and take in what has been said. It may be helpful for a member of staff to share a cup of tea with them. For out-patients check that they have a means of getting home safely, perhaps someone to drive them. If they are going home alone, ensure that they feel able to take this on. If not, arrange for a family member or friend to pick them up. Warn them that further feelings may appear later as the news sinks in.

Follow-up

Always offer a follow-up meeting for those who have attended as out-patients. Those on the ward will be visited frequently by the members of the multidisciplinary team so there will be ample opportunity to see them again and discuss their further concerns. Whenever I have broken bad news to someone at home it has usually been along with the community nurse specialist. We then arrange that she will come back and see the patient a few days later to follow up any questions he may have. He can also contact her by phone before then should he feel the need.

The following is an example of a breaking bad news scenario:

Althea transcript

Althea has been admitted to the hospice at the request of her community nurse specialist. Over the weekend, Althea found that her legs were going numb, tingling and weak and that she was becoming incontinent of urine. Her husband called out the deputising doctor on call service three times. She was told she had a urinary tract infection and given antibiotics; later she was given quinine for cramps. In the hospice, which is attached to the local hospital, she had an MRI scan which showed that she had spinal cord compression causing her weak legs and incontinence. I, along with the ward junior doctor, Anna, and the ward sister, Jenny, are seeing Althea and her husband, Winston, together. Winston is wearing a dark suit and tie and standing anxiously in the corner of the room.

Louis: Hallo, Althea – and you must be Winston; we've not met
    before.

Winston: Hi.

Louis: Anna has been telling me about what's been happening to you last weekend – it seems a lot's been going on.

Althea: [nods] It was a complete nightmare; you have no idea.

Louis: I imagine it must have been very frightening.

Althea: Yes – and we couldn't get anybody to do anything about it. The deputising doctors just kept fobbing us off. They wouldn't listen. Thank God there was a bed in the hospice.

Louis: I guess it must have been difficult for you, too, Winston; you had your two children to look after as well as Althea being unwell.

Winston: Yeah – and she would keep trying to get up and help when I told her to stay in bed, and then she'd trip and fall. But, Althea's mother was able to come and stay, so that helped a lot.

Louis: And how are you feeling today, Althea?

Althea: Scared; I want to know what's going to happen next. I mean, will I be paralysed?... I couldn't bear that... And I hate this catheter.

Jenny: We talked about that earlier today, didn't we, and we agreed it was worthwhile temporarily.

Althea: Yes, I know. It's just so undignified.

Anna: I explained to Althea and Winston about the reasons for the MRI scan – to see if there is any compression of the spinal cord.

Louis: And that's why we're here now – to talk about the results of the scan.

Winston: So what did you find?

Louis: First, it shows what we knew already – that there is cancer in the spine.

Althea: Yes, I was expecting that.

Louis: ...Second, it does show that the cancer is compressing your spinal cord...[silence]...and that's why your legs are weak and you're wetting yourself.

Althea: [looking frozen] I don't quite understand.

Louis: ...The nerves to your legs and bladder aren't working properly because of the pressure on them.

Althea: Oh God...that's what we feared...[begins to cry; Winston holds her hand]...[silence].

Louis: What's happening, Althea?

Althea: I was just thinking about what this means...it's losing control... I hate not being in control... It's so scary...

Winston: What can we do then, doctor? Anna was talking about further treatment to shrink the cancer.

Louis: Althea, I know you're upset. Are you OK with me talking about your treatment? [Althea nods]...First then, we'll start you on steroids – these will help by reducing the swelling in the spinal canal and so reducing the pressure on the spinal cord; that can help the weak legs and bladder trouble.

Althea: Well, at least that's something.

Winston: Are there any problems with taking steroids? That's not what athletes take for body building is it?

Louis: That's a different type of steroid. The one we're prescribing, dexamethasone, doesn't have that effect. In the short term, steroids don't usually have serious problems. They may, in fact, make you feel better – and they often increase your appetite.

Winston: And Anna was mentioning radiotherapy.

Louis: Yes. If you agree, we'll arrange for you to go to the radiotherapy department at St Philip's Hospital today for assessment.

Althea: Today? Does it have to be today?

Louis: Yes, it is important. The more quickly you have the radiotherapy, the more likely it is to prevent further problems.

Althea: Further problems? What does that mean?

Louis: The radiotherapy is to prevent the weakness of the legs increasing.

Winston: And will it do that?

Louis: Although there isn't a complete guarantee, usually
       radiotherapy is successful as long as the treatment is given
       without delay...

Althea: [starts to cry] Oh my God... Oh my God...it has to
        work... Please God that it will work.

Louis: I can see how distressing this is for you, Althea. And I'm
       sorry that I'm having to give you such a lot of
       information – it must be difficult to take it all in.

Althea: [crying] Just do it doctor – I must do everything I can.
        I've got Rachel and Jack to think of... God, I feel I've let
        them down. I must get on my feet again ... I will be able
        to drive again, won't I?

Louis: It will depend on the effect of the radiotherapy. As I said,
       it usually stops the weakness and bladder trouble getting
       any worse and not infrequently it can improve the
       strength of the legs and bladder control.

[Althea sits silently, quietly crying, and holding tightly to
       Winston's hand]

Winston: Well, at least there is some treatment.

Althea: But what are we going to tell Rachel and Jack?

Winston: We'll just say Mum's got to be in hospital for a few
         days and you'll be home soon.

Althea: But I might not be at this rate.

Jenny: Many of the parents we talk to worry about how to deal
       with this. They've often found it helpful to talk to our
       social worker, Debbie, who has worked a lot with
       children. If you like, I can ask her to look in after this
       meeting and chat to you.

Althea: Please, yes...

Louis: It's natural to think about all that this may mean to you in
       your lives, but I would suggest that we take this one step
       at a time. Our first job is to contact the radiotherapy
       department and arrange for you to be seen by them.

Althea: Will I have to stay there?

Anna: It's possible, but not certain. Once I've phoned them I
      should be able to tell you one way or the other. It's
      possible they may just give you a single dose of

radiotherapy in which case you could come straight back afterwards.

Althea: I hope so; I'd prefer to be here. It feels safer than a hospital.

Louis: Is there anything else either of you would like to ask?

Althea: No. But my mind is in a blur, so something may come up later.

Anna: When I come back later you'll have had some time to think over what we've been discussing – we can talk further then.

Winston: OK. Let's get her across to St Philip's as quickly as possible.

Louis: A lot of what we've discussed today has been about the scan results and your treatment. I imagine you will have a lot of feelings about what's been said. I'll come and see you again when you get back from having your radiotherapy and we can continue talking.

The above example gives a flavour of the process of breaking bad news in circumstances of some medical urgency. In an actual situation, the conversation might well last longer if issues such as talking to their children are explored further. It can be seen that the giving of information necessarily forms a major part of the discussion in this case. Emotional issues are acknowledged and touched on, but, given the circumstances, have to be followed up in more depth later. Note, too, that three members of staff take part. This is obviously the best way of ensuring good interdisciplinary communication. After such a meeting, it would be usual for the staff taking part to debrief – discuss practicalities of management and share any feelings about emotionally taxing aspects of the discussion, a good way of informally supporting each other. Although I, as the consultant, was the main person speaking to Althea on this occasion, it could equally well be other members of staff instead.

The scene now moves to the next afternoon and we are meeting again.

Louis: Hallo… Anna's told me you've had your radiotherapy. How are you both feeling today?

Althea: Well, relieved that it's over…and nervous – wondering if the treatment will work.

Louis: Wondering if it will work?

Althea: Yes... I mean it has to. I can't bear to think that it might not.

Louis: It feels unbearable to think that?

Althea: [after a silence] It's my children I keep thinking about. They need me. I *have* to get better for their sake. But I feel so helpless... God I hate this bloody cancer...

Louis: ...So, a mixture of feelings – helplessness and anger.

Althea: It's so unfair. I'm young – why should it be me that gets cancer? It's the story of my life. One disaster after another. There was that miscarriage...and my brother dying in that hit-and-run car accident. Maybe I'm being punished.

Winston: Come on Thea, you mustn't think like that. We'll get through this.

Louis: Althea, I want to acknowledge that you've obviously had many crises to deal with, but I wonder, right now, where in your body do you notice your feelings?

Althea: [after a moment's silence, she puts her hand on her chest] It's mainly here, a sort of aching soreness, but then...[she moves her hand down to her solar plexus]... I feel like I've been kicked in the gut as well.

Louis: If these feelings and sensations had a voice, what might they be saying?

Althea: [begins to cry]...Oh, I feel such a lot of sorrow for my children and for Winston – to have to put them through this.

Winston: It's all right Thea, we're with you.

Louis: Althea, it sounds very compassionate what you're saying.

Althea: [tearfully] Well I love them, I'd do anything for them.

Louis: Maybe you can do something for them.

Althea: What do you mean?

Louis: Well, you were thinking in terms of all the things you couldn't do at the moment. But my guess is that Rachel and Jack just want to be with you right now, maybe talk to you, perhaps read a story together. Those are things

you *can* do together. I imagine you would have plenty of
ideas along those lines.

Althea: Yes... I see...

And the conversation continues. In this scene, counselling skills are used
more than in the previous meeting to pick up on feelings, and Althea
returns to her ongoing concerns about her family. I concentrate mostly on
talking with Althea, but as the discussion continues, I would turn to
Winston as well for his reactions and watch for the interactions between
them. Althea is experiencing feelings of being a victim and seeing the situation as a catastrophe, unsurprisingly given what's happened. Note how,
by focusing on her bodily feelings, she is able to get in touch with her
emotions. I acknowledge and respect her feelings and her need to grieve
her losses, and we then begin to move into a more resourceful framing of
her predicament. Thinking about what *can* be done helps to re-empower
her and move out of identification with being a victim.

CHAPTER 7

Working with Emotions

SURVIVAL REACTIONS

Many of our emotions are intimately connected with survival. In biological terms these are the fight, flight and freeze reactions (Levine 1997). The first two are very familiar, but the third is, perhaps, less well known. And yet, we have only to look at the animal world to see these dramas played out daily. A cheetah chases a young impala, the hunter pursuing its fleeing prey. But:

> At the moment of contact...the young impala falls to the ground, surrendering to its impending death. Yet, it may be uninjured. The stone-still animal is not pretending to be dead. It has instinctively entered an altered state of consciousness shared by all mammals when death appears imminent. (Levine 1997, pp.15–16)

This last-ditch strategy has two purposes: playing possum just occasionally allows escape, and the animal is in an altered state where no pain is felt. The explorer, David Livingstone, attested to this when he survived being mauled by a lion – he described going into a dream-like state in which he experienced no fear or pain (Chatwin 1987, p.271).

Unsurprisingly, the prospect of dying activates these survival responses. We see the fight response in a patient's determination to fight for life, in his anger and aggression. Flight manifests as fear, anxiety, panic attacks, restlessness, agitation, ceaseless activity, or leaving the hospice or hospital before treatment has been arranged. Freezing may show itself in lethargy, depression, apathy, staying in bed, sleeping all the time or dissociation.

There is a further twist to this. If an animal that has gone into the freeze response escapes death, the physiological hyperarousal still pertains and needs to be discharged. One important way mammals do this is through shivering. We humans often suppress our emotional responses. However, they do not go away. They are engraved in the emotional brain and return as traumatic reactions including depression, panic attacks or nightmares. A trauma trap is created where triggering threats and emotional responses cycle endlessly without resolution. When, then, patients complain of shivering and restlessness, this may be their body attempting to discharge the pent up energies of a past trauma. Aspirin and diazepam might mask the symptoms but they won't address the fundamental issue.

It is clear, then, that much work in palliative care is around managing these threat responses, in providing a milieu where patients and family can feel safe enough.

APPROACHING EMOTIONS

There are a number of questions that can be useful to ask, whatever the emotion being expressed. This, however, is not to be done mechanically by rote but rather in context when the right moment presents itself:

- Tell me about what you are feeling.
- What brought on these feelings?
- Do you remember times in the past when you felt this way?
- As you notice the feelings, what sensations are you experiencing in your body?
- If your feelings had a voice, what would they say?
- Are there any images that you associate with these feelings?

Beware of saying you understand how the patient feels. You may think you do, but it's easy to get it wrong. Barasch (1993, p.333) describes recovering from an operation for thyroid cancer. A visitor looked in when he was having a bad day. As he tried to tell her in a rough post-operative voice how horrible it felt to have his thyroid taken away, 'her baffled look suddenly resolved into an expression of empathy. "I know how you feel," she said. "I once got this really *terrible* haircut, and there was nothing I could do…"'

ANGER

In a way it is surprising that anger isn't more overt in the dying. It can be, of course, but upbringing and culture are potent restraining factors for many. More prevalent is partially suppressed anger which makes itself known in many ways: irritation, grumbling, brooding, self-destructiveness, bitterness, coldness and so on. It's my impression that anger in patients and relatives causes more staff disquiet than any other emotion – they may feel personally threatened. So much of our time as clinicians is spent listening to dying people and supporting them and one of the paybacks, like it or not, is that we are often praised and thanked for what we do, and rightly so. But, should an angry, complaining, manipulative patient appear on the scene, then staff stress levels rise rapidly as witnessed by their expression of their disquiet at ward meetings.

Is there a cancer-prone personality, one in which anger is suppressed? Some studies have suggested as much (LeShan 1994) though other research disputes this. Whatever the truth of it, there is an important caveat here. Patients may already feel they are somehow deficient physically, that it was their fault that they developed cancer. Their guilt may then be compounded by the thought that their previous psychological state might have brought on their illness, as some alternative practitioners promulgate. This unnecessary self-shaming, at times a re-evocation of childhood parental shamings, is destructive and unhelpful, especially in the last weeks of their life. Rather, counselling support needs to emphasise self-acceptance.

Anger may be manifested at anybody and anything, even though it originates in the cancer diagnosis. It is as though this discovery acts as a trigger, re-energising unhealed memories and breaking down the barriers containing previously suppressed emotions. So, clinical staff, the hospice, the hospital, the treatment, family members, friends, lovers, enemies, places of work, the NHS and God, among others, may all be targets, a displacement of the rage the patient feels at her body for letting her down. Of course, her anger may be justified. She may have received poor treatment. Her place of work may have dismissed her unfairly. Her husband may have had an affair. All this needs to be acknowledged. Nevertheless, underneath the anger is pain, pain that may be so unbearable that she doesn't want to let it into awareness, pain at the prospect of losing her life, her loved ones, her career.

Unresolved anger, in the form of chronic resentment, blame or hatred will have a noxious effect on an individual's life and his relationships. It is like an acid that eats away at his soul. The character of Gollum from *The Lord of the Rings* exemplifies this: he cares only for his 'precious', the ring of power that slowly corrupts any who wear it. When Bilbo Baggins takes this ring, the twisted Gollum shrieks out in a voice filled with hatred and despair, '…thief! Baggins! We hates it…we hates it for ever!' (Tolkien 1966, p.98, first published 1937).

Having said this, other people use their anger constructively, whether it is in their determination to battle with their cancer, to fight for the chemotherapy they need that is not available on the NHS or to be able to get home again despite having become paraplegic. Anger, then, is of itself simply a natural energy. It is how we use it – for good or ill – that makes the difference.

Inability to contain anger may also be a feature of psychological illnesses with organic features, such as psychoses, alcoholism and bipolar disorders. This may need treatment with psychotropic drugs as a substitute for the loss of normal inhibitory controls.

So how can we work with anger effectively? A common and understandable staff defence mechanism is to blame the patient. However, assigned the role of scapegoat, he can become even more isolated than before. In turn this may aggravate his already antisocial behaviour, and a downward spiral of deteriorating relationships ensues. To avoid this, a different, and more demanding, approach is needed, one that takes the patient's anger seriously:

- Take time before the encounter to discuss with colleagues how best to approach the meeting and what your position will be. This will also help prevent the situation where the patient or family give contradictory messages to different staff members, which could potentially split the team.

- Listen with an open mind and without interrupting. So often, this is what the patient has not had. Her grievance has not been taken seriously. The very act of paying attention as she expresses his feelings may, in itself, help to contain her anger.

- Find some way of empathising with the patient. You may not agree with him, but you can still say, 'I can see how upset you are about this', or, 'I'm so sorry that you have had such a difficult time with this'.

- Be on the lookout for what's beneath the anger. Her fury at the unsuccessful treatment may hide a terror of dying.

- The patient or relative may be completely justified in feeling angry, as with a delay in diagnosis. While you can empathise with their story, it is, however, important not to take sides – you have, after all, only heard one side of the story.

- Some patients are so taken over by rage that they jump from subject to subject – the delay in diagnosis, his pain-killers don't work, he wants a second opinion, his son has crashed his car, he is in big financial trouble if he doesn't go back to work, his wife isn't visiting and so on. When his catharsis has moderated his anger, there may be an opportunity gently to bring him back to the original topic. You can agree with him to return to the other issues later.

- If you or your team have made a mistake, then in general it's best to say so and apologise. Mostly, patients are only looking for a recognition of their grievance. The only exception to this is if litigation is possible. In this case an expression of regret at what has happened can still be given, but no comment on liability can be made as this must be dealt with by your defence union.¹ If in doubt, an informal discussion with your union will clarify the way forward.

- As far as possible, avoid confrontation, both in the way you speak and in your body language – avoid staring, and speak quietly, for example. Even if you feel upset at some unjust accusation, argument will simply tend to escalate the tension by polarising the relationship between you – as far as the patient is concerned, you have joined 'them' and so are no longer to be trusted. Later, when she has said what she wanted to say and calmed down, she may be more open to discussion.

- However, it's important not to cave in and agree with everything the patient or family says. You will have a view on their complaints and, after they have had their say, it may be necessary to state this. For example, the patient who insists that he wants only one particular nurse to look after him because all the rest are no good will need to be told that the nurses work as

1   Malpractice indemnity insurers.

a team, sharing duties, and his demand is not the way the ward works. A relative who insists on being told what is wrong with the patient may need to be informed that the patient does not wish her to be told. This setting of boundaries is not meant to be draconian; rather it can provide security in a crisis situation. Those involved know where they stand. Speaking your truth quietly, without aggression or attributing blame, has its own power.

- Occasionally, patients or relatives will not accept what a junior member of staff has to say and it may become necessary to involve a more senior staff member. This is usually successful, more because of its symbolic value than any disparity in approach. It is an important message to patients that the senior clinician backs what the junior had to say. It demonstrates a unity of approach.

- Take time later to talk through with a colleague or friend how you felt about the meeting.

ANXIETY

While it is important to look out for organic causes of anxiety such as thyrotoxicosis or glucocorticosteroid medication, mostly, psychological causes pertain to anxiety. There is one condition that falls between these two camps – breathlessness. This symptom is intimately linked with anxiety. Shortness of breath from, for example, lung cancer brings with it the possibility of suffocation and hence induces intense anxiety. The attendant adrenaline output increases the body's metabolic rate dramatically, including the need for oxygen. The brain signals to the body to breathe more but the respiratory muscles are already overburdened. Reduced oxygen and increased carbon dioxide in the blood aggravate the breathlessness, resulting in yet more anxiety and a vortex of worsening symptoms ensues.

Breathlessness can also be a psychosomatic symptom stemming from anxiety with no lung pathology. Indeed, panic attacks can present as acute hyperventilation. Perhaps the first time we felt this combination of fear and suffocation was during labour. Some degree of hypoxia is common, especially during the second stage of labour when it is associated with intense compression by the contracting uterus. Indeed, one sign of foetal distress in the womb due to lack of oxygen is respiratory gasping. It is no wonder that so many babies cry when they are born. It is more than the need to breathe – it is also an expression of their emotional stress, which may include fear. While we do not remember this consciously as adults, our unconscious retains an atavistic impression that may be re-evoked when our breathing is threatened.

In palliative care, anxiety may be related to the following:

- physical suffering – such as severe pain or breathlessness
- loss – of health, body parts, mental faculties, sexuality, mobility, control, status, beauty, family and friends, work
- re-evocation of unhealed past memories
- the prospect of death – extinction of life, a painful death or going to hell.

It is quite likely that the patient will be on some form of tranquillising medication already, but this need not interfere with a counselling approach as long as he is alert enough to talk. Indeed, by softening the intensity of his emotional reactions, it can make it possible for him to talk about issues too frightening to face before.

Anxious patients are in emergency mode. It is important, therefore, to build a relationship that feels safe enough for them. I say 'safe enough' because it will, of course, be necessary to address their fears, but in a context where they do not feel out of control. They are like ships tossed by a stormy sea of emotions; they are in need of a protective harbour where they can look at the storm without being overwhelmed by it. This is important – for it is when the patient begins to face what he fears that the fear, paradoxically, can begin, however slowly, to dissolve.

The Buddhist nun, Pema Chödrön, describes a striking example of this. A friend of hers had nightmares of 'running through a huge dark building pursued by hideous monsters…she'd wake up screaming.' Pema asked her what the monsters looked like. She didn't know. But, the next time the nightmare took place, in her dream, she stopped fleeing and turned to face these fiends. 'It took tremendous courage, and her heart was pounding.' They leapt up and down but didn't come any nearer. She studied them and saw that 'they appeared less like monsters and more like two-dimensional drawings in comic books.' Gradually they disappeared. The nightmares never returned (Chödrön 1997, pp.28–29). The key phrase here is: 'It took tremendous courage.' This is really true, especially if we are considering illness, suffering or loss. But, often, it is our *perceptions* that become the monsters, perceptions that may be the offspring of our lifelong, secret fears – of being eternally alone, of falling into darkness forever, of suffocation, of hell – which attach themselves to, and darkly colour, the knowledge that we are soon to die. However, while the prospect of death may be very frightening, terminally ill people can and do move out of their fear and do grow to accept their ending. Not infrequently, the moment of dying can actually be profoundly peaceful.

Not only is anxiety very distressing but it can also impair thinking, which will affect the reflective approach needed in counselling. Hence the use of relaxation and visualisation exercises can be helpful in reducing anxiety and its associated physiological arousal. These have been described in detail in Chapter 5. If the patient uses a visualisation exercise, this can become a 'safe place' for her, an image that she can return to mentally at any time if she feels distressed. Furthermore, as already described, visualisations can be used to work on emotional issues.

The following are practical pointers in working with anxious patients:

- Giving a message that you are not put off or fazed by what the patient has to say can be reassuring to him. You are providing the safe containment that he desperately needs and is unable to provide for himself. So, stillness, unhurriedness, alert listening and empathic interventions will all contribute to this.

- Anxious people look at the world through disaster-tinted glasses. While it is true they have genuine cause for anxiety because of their cancer diagnosis, this may spill over so that they feel every symptom means they are about to die, that the treatments won't work, that they will be in agony. Hence a careful assessment of their unrealistic catastrophe scenarios and the consequent insight that they are not valid may help to reduce their fear. Some people find it helpful to hear of studies demonstrating, for example, successful pain control, and these can be quoted to back up the point.

- False reassurance is not helpful, though families may try and persuade you to give it. One woman spent hours holding her partner and reassuring him that he was all right despite the fact that he had an advanced and progressive cancer. She tried to persuade the staff to do the same and had great difficulty in seeing what was plainly before her eyes: that he was anxious and not reassured and kept asking staff members to tell him the truth.

- Anxious patients may wish to hold your hand as you talk with them. While this is not usual in counselling, it is commonplace in palliative care and is often much appreciated as a gesture of support.

- Touch-based complementary therapies such as massage, aromatherapy and reflexology may have a profoundly calming effect which will support counselling interventions. Indeed, some patients like to talk about their concerns during a massage – they feel safe enough to do so.

- Anxious patients who hyperventilate can be referred to the physiotherapist for breathing retraining exercises.

- Some patients have intense anxieties around religious and spiritual issues. Here, the chaplain can have an important role, either from the perspective of spiritual counsel, or as a mediator of religious rituals. One terminally ill man felt he could not be forgiven for his sins and was convinced the Devil was waiting for him. He was Catholic and the chaplain administered the sacrament of reconciliation. The ritual spoke to him where words alone could not and his anxiety faded away with his absolution.

DEPRESSION

From the perspective of the medical model, depression is thought of as a disease brought on by such factors as genetic predisposition or depletion of brain neurotransmitters (Puri, Laking and Treasaden 1996, pp.168–70). However, everyone experiences a mild form of depression from time to time, only it's given different names: 'the blues' or 'feeling down' or 'miserable'. Indeed, there is no clear dividing line between normal and pathological depressed mood. Similarly, there is no test to diagnose depression. Instead, clinical criteria used are based on expert psychiatric opinion. These, at least, gives a reference point for assessing significant depression and the place of medical treatment. The following are features that may occur (numbers in brackets refer to the American Psychiatric Association (2000) criteria):

- mood

    o depressed mood (1)

    o diurnal variation of mood, lower in the mornings and improved by evening

- o sadness and tearfulness (1)
- o hopelessness
- o feelings of guilt and worthlessness (7)
- o emptiness (1)
- o anxiety
- o irritability
- o anhedonia – loss of interest and enjoyment in activities (2)
- physical state
  - o weight loss or gain with corresponding appetite changes (3)
  - o insomnia or hypersomnia (4)
  - o psychomotor agitation or retardation (5)
  - o self-neglect
  - o loss of energy (6)
  - o depressed appearance
- thinking
  - o reduced ability to concentrate and think (8)
  - o memory difficulties due to poor concentration
  - o indecisiveness (8)
  - o thoughts of death and suicide (9)
  - o cognitive triad of a negative view of self, the outer world and the future (Beck 1989)
- other
  - o social withdrawal
  - o masked depression due to somatisation, cultural factors or dementia
  - o in severe depression, psychotic features such as paranoid delusions.

The Diagnostic and Statistical Manual or DSM IV-TR (American Psychiatric Association 2000) lists nine features which form their diagnostic criteria for major depression (numbered 1–9 in the list above). At least five of these should be present for at least a fortnight to make a diagnosis. Palliative care patients, however, do not fit so easily into these criteria. This is because many of the features specified such as weight loss or loss of energy may be due to the cancer itself. Endicott (1984) tried to make allowance for this by substituting alternative criteria where needed. Thus, instead of change of weight, she put in, 'tearfulness and depressed appearance'; for sleep changes, she substituted, 'social withdrawal or decreased talkativeness'; for loss of energy, 'brooding self-pity, or pessimism'; for thinking difficulties, 'cannot be cheered up, doesn't smile, no response to good news or funny situations' (p.2247).

In practice, by far the most useful question is, very simply: 'Are you depressed?' This needs to be followed, of course, by suitable enquiry as to the depression's severity and around feelings of suicide, which will be discussed shortly. It may, too, be obvious prior to any discussion that someone is depressed. This is not only about they way she looks – the expressionless face, the slow movements and so on – but also the 'feel' of the patient, what you pick up in your countertransference.

While major depression is usually treated by antidepressants, we are still left with the very common depressive reaction to terminal illness, so common that it can often be seen as a normal response to an overwhelming crisis. In psychotherapeutic terms, depression is often considered to be a result of inturned anger, or of unresolved grief and, certainly, both these scenarios are frequently a part of facing dying. Remember, too, the fight/flight/freeze triad of threat reactions referred to at the beginning of this chapter. In some ways, depression has features that parallel the freeze reaction. Pursuing this analogy further, it can therefore likewise be seen as a primal survival mechanism in the face of a life-threatening illness that cannot be fought off or run away from. How can this be? One aspect of depression is its *blunting* of emotions and lack of physical energy. It is often described as a grey fog. If this numbing blanket were to be lifted suddenly, the depressed person could experience the full force of his psychological pain at knowing he is dying. Depression itself can be intensely distressing, but the alternative may seem, to the sufferer, even worse. However, this is a two-edged sword for, while most of us will find that our mood lifts again after some setback, those who are facing the prospect of dying may, instead, sometimes spiral down into a black despair even more anguishing than the original pain and needing both pharmacological and psychological support.

In practice, other features of the survival triad come through too, so it is common to see agitation and irritability as part of a depressive reaction, as if the psyche cycles between fight, flight or freeze as the best strategy.

Talking with depressed people can be difficult because of their lack of response. Questions are answered briefly or not at all. They may look away and seem uninterested. It feels as though there is a wall between you, which, in psychological terms, there is. How is this barrier to be worked with? First, as always, it is important to get alongside the patient, to enter her world, in this case of blankness, greyness, no energy, feeling depressed, perhaps wanting to die. Ask her, then, to describe this very experience, what it feels like in her body. Does she have any images she associates with the feeling? A famous example of this is Winston Churchill, who described times when he felt depressed as black dog days. Be interested in how the patient is at this moment rather than trying to get her to snap out of it.

Look for very subtle signs. She may not talk much, but she may, perhaps, sigh from time to time. She may hold her hands protectively in front of her stomach. She may turn away from you. She may shake her head. She may cry silently and with no expression. Consider commenting on what you have noticed, however trivial it might seem: 'I notice that, when I asked you when your depression started, you crossed your arms over your stomach. I wonder what was happening then?' You can comment directly about her silence in the same way.

Forming a therapeutic alliance with a depressed patient may be difficult but is vitally important. One useful question is to ask is if she would like to be free of the depression. This, unlike other enquiries, may evoke a strong response. She may say of course she does; it is intensely distressing and she would give anything to be rid of it. If she can then realise that you are genuinely an ally and wanting to help her, this may remove a few bricks from the defensive wall she has built around herself.

Depression in the dying is often about disempowerment. They feel there is no point in trying since the cancer is advancing and resistant to treatment and this casts a pallid gloom over their whole life, including the parts where they do retain control. One way of working with this is to consider, too, what they *can* do, to look at unfinished business that they want to, and can realistically, finish – working with where their energy is. The key here is that word 'realistic'. If asked their goals, patients will often start with aims that are out of reach and this calls for negotiation to find a pragmatic compromise. I recall one man who was paraplegic from spinal cancer insisted on buying a new car despite being warned that he would never be able to drive it, and this is what happened. By contrast, another woman, with the same condition, decided that she wanted to continue running the firm she owned. She fully accepted she was paraplegic. She was also very determined. While she adapted to a wheelchair existence, she arranged to have her car converted to manual controls, learnt the skills required and was able to drive on the motorway to and from work. I am not suggesting this as an example for everyone, but rather that we worked with what *she* wanted and kept it practical.

In counselling clients with depression, it is important not to try to rescue them from their symptom, not to try to make it magically go away. Rather, be prepared, when they are ready, to address it, explore it, understand its origins, even if this may be painful. It is when the message of the depression, what it is there for, has been heard that healing can begin.

Depression is a symptom that is usually resistant to rapid change, which contrasts with those who are feeling anxious or angry, who may sometimes feel temporarily much better after even one session for having talked through their issues. This depressive inertia isn't necessarily an issue in those who are not dying, since there is time to work with it, but it is a major dilemma in palliative care, since these patients may only have days or weeks to live. The usual approach taken is to try to alleviate their distress, since it would seem very harsh for them to spend their few remaining days alive suffering from the often intense anguish of depression. Attempts are often made to resolve depression with drugs. Antidepressants take two weeks to begin to work and so should only be used in those who will live longer than this time. Amphetamines can be used as psychostimulants that lift mood within a few days – they are more commonly used for this purpose in the USA than in the British Isles.

Two other factors help here. One is the intensive staff input usual in hospices. The second is that most depressed patients have features of sadness, anxiety or anger, emotions that have broken through their depressive wall. It is then sometimes possible to work with the energies released by these feelings and to find a way in towards their source.

A number of patients remain in their depressed state, whether through being unable to find a way out of their grey world, or through choice. This is a difficult issue for those working in palliative care. It would be wonderful to be able to render every depressed person alert and happy. The reality may be more complex. For example, it is too much to expect a person who has been depressed for decades, has a history of childhood trauma and repeated suicide attempts, to suddenly become un-depressed in the last two weeks of his life. It *can* happen but it can't be legislated for.

In such cases the way in which hospice patients are made to feel secure comes to the fore. The nursing care provided, baths, massages, symptom control, quietness, volunteers to sit with them, music they like, open visiting, all give a message of support. Often, patients are taking powerful pain-relieving drugs or tranquillisers and these will reduce their awareness of their depressed feelings. Some will opt to sleep most of the time. Finally, as they approach death, they may slip into a coma.

SUICIDAL FEELINGS

The life instinct is so powerful that, even in the face of a terminal illness, many patients will still search for remission or even cure. Suicidal feelings, which might be called the death instinct, are also common. It is only humans who have the self-awareness to realise that they can take their own lives, but their motivation may be varied. It may be:

- to escape unbearable pain or other physical symptoms
- to escape psychological pain such as depression
- as part of the syndrome of clinical depression
- a response to loss of physical abilities – paralysis, loss of speech, incontinence
- a considered anticipatory response to a progressive fatal illness such as motor neurone disease
- a wish to make others close to the suicidal person suffer – 'Look what you made me do, it's your fault'

- the ultimate form of self-destructiveness in people with extreme self-hatred – 'I'm worthless, the world would be better off if I were dead'

- a primitive, instinctive regression – patients who take to their bed, refuse to eat or drink and become mute

- sacrificial – the person who gives up his life for another.

It might be thought that actual suicide would be a frequent occurrence in the dying. In the five palliative care units in which I have worked, it was a very rare occurrence. Possible reasons for this include:

- the intensive care input provided by palliative care services, including psychological support

- the instinctive wish to live as long as possible

- the discovery that it is still possible for life to be satisfying and enjoyable even if death is not far off

- the belief among some patients that suicide is wrong, for example for religious reasons

- not wanting to cause distress to their family

- a fear of not succeeding in a suicide attempt and waking up worse off than before.

Thoughts about dying have a symbolic dimension. Whenever we pass through any life transition such as birth, puberty or parenthood, this involves a metaphorical dying to what came before. This 'little death' imperative gestates in our unconscious, waiting to come into our awareness at the appropriate time. It is the same for a terminal illness. There is a calling from our unconscious – it is time for us to go. Such thoughts are a normal part of dying, but they may be re-interpreted. 'I want to die' can become translated into a literalistic acting out: 'I'm going to kill myself'. It may help here to ask: 'Who wants to die?' You may then find that it is one aspect of the patient's personality, such as the inner Victim, who has suffered previously and whose distress has been reactivated by the terminal illness.

It may also be useful to ask what is underneath this wish for self-destruction – for this may also be a defence, hiding a deeper pain that the patient cannot face. One woman, deeply in love with her husband who was dying, talked in detail about how she would commit suicide after he died. She could not contemplate the thought of being without him, who was, to her, her whole life. But behind this was an unhappy and unloved childhood – she had given her husband the love she could not share with her parents and his dying re-evoked these memories. Interestingly, she did not commit suicide afterwards.

In assessing suicide risk, ask first about thoughts of self-harm. Some fear this will put ideas into the patient's head. This is not so. If they have not thought of suicide it is because they have no need to. If they have been thinking about suicide it will more likely be a relief for them to be able to share the burden of their feelings. It may seem a difficult topic to broach but, nevertheless, it is a vital one in the assessment of severity of depression. It can be approached gradually. Each of the following questions is a step more direct than its predecessor and the appropriate one can be chosen depending what you feel the patient will be able to accept:

- 'You have been talking about feeling depressed; I was wondering whether you have times of feeling that there's no point to life?'
- 'Do you ever feel that life is not worth living?'
- 'Do you ever feel you wish you were dead?'
- 'Do you ever feel like ending it all?'
- 'Have you considered taking your own life?'
- 'Have you thought about methods of suicide?'

Gauging the likelihood of suicide is not easy. Even the most experienced practitioner will be mistaken at times. The Samaritans have used a scoring system which provides a practical, if approximate, assessment of risk (Vining 1995):

The risk scores derived from Table 7.1 are as follows:

- Imminent danger. Do not leave alone   7–8 in part A

  20 or more in total

- High risk. Arrange another meeting soon   14–19
- Moderate risk. Another meeting should be fixed   6–11
- Slight risk. Hear the person out and let him or her go unless there are reasons to meet again   0 in part A
  1–5 in total.

Table 7.1 Samaritans' suicide risk assessment (Vining 1995)

SCORING TABLE USED TO ASSESS RISK OF SUICIDE	
CHOOSE ONE FIGURE TO SCORE SUICIDE PLAN	
Chief indicator of immediate risk	
Imminent sudden death	8
Imminent slow method of suicide	7
Future sudden death planned	6
Future slow method of suicide planned	5
Planning suicide 'gamble'	4
Planning suicidal gesture	3
Definite suicidal thoughts but has no plan	2
Toying vaguely with idea of suicide	1
No suicidal thoughts	0
ADD POINTS FOR EVERY RELEVANT ITEM	
Mostly the long-term factors	
Previous suicidal acts or gestures	</=4
Recent broken relationship. Isolation. Rejection	3 (each)
No hope. Loss of faith	3 (each)
Depressive illness	3
Dependence on alcohol or drugs	2
Possession of means of suicide	2
Putting affairs in order	2
Over 60. Male. Ill. Chronic pain	1 (each)

Note that 'illness' is a given for all palliative care patients and indeed rates of suicide are known to be raised in those with cancer, especially in the terminal phase (Breitbart, Chochinov and Passik 2004, p.755). Psychopathologies, such as psychoses, also carry a higher risk. 'Chronic pain' is present in about three-quarters of those with terminal malignant disease; it is understandable that its severity, if untreated, might become unbearable and drive a person to take his own life.

Threat of suicide is obviously a concern for palliative care clinicians. However, their responsibility is a careful assessment of risk, provision of treatment by a doctor if needed, and referral to clinical support services, including the psychiatric team if necessary. It is possible, despite these precautions, that a patient, or his relative, might attempt suicide. This, however, should not be seen as a reflection on the care provided. It may be deeply painful for those who have worked with the patient, and they may *feel* responsible, but, it must be stressed, it is not their fault.

What action, then, can we take in dealing with a patient with suicidal ideation?

- Use the counselling skills already described to explore how the suicidal thinking came about. The patient may well feel very isolated and hence your listening empathically is time well spent. You are giving him a counter-message telling him he is not alone and that he is worth listening to. He may find it a huge relief to voice his thoughts.

- Some patients feel suicidal because of continual severe pain or other symptoms such as breathlessness. It is obvious that good symptom control is what is needed here.

- Are there other precipitating factors such as family conflict or alcohol abuse where support such as family meetings or Alcoholics Anonymous may help?

- Is the patient clinically depressed? If so, she will probably require antidepressant medication.

- Is there a significant risk of self-harm? In-patients can be closely monitored by the ward staff. For out-patients, their GP must be contacted so that she can continue clinical responsibility for their care. It may be necessary to involve psychiatric support services too – an early out-patient appointment or a visit from a community psychiatric nurse. It can help to ask the patient to promise not to harm herself until you see her again. This gives her a goal to aim for.

- Close follow-up by the palliative care community nurse specialist will provide further support. He can liaise with the GP, psychiatric team or hospice staff if he has concerns.

- Where possible, involve the family in providing support – particularly if the patient lives alone – by visiting him.

- If there are severe mental health problems such as a psychotic depression or a bipolar illness with marked mood swings, then psychiatric referral is urgent. It can be difficult to decide whether such in-patients should be cared for on the psychiatric ward where there is mental health expertise, or on the palliative care ward where there is proficiency in terminal care. The level of physical needs usually decides the matter, since psychiatric wards are not set up for intensive palliative care.

- Remember that, as patients begin to respond to antidepressants after a fortnight or so, their energy levels may increase while their mood is still low, putting them at a temporary further risk of carrying out a suicide threat.

GUILT AND SHAME

Guilt is the feeling associated with the belief that we have done wrong, whether by commission or omission. Shame is the feeling that we are wrong or bad or deficient in ourselves. These emotions may at times serve a purpose. We may have good reason to feel guilty if we have betrayed our own inner values. Guilt will tend to look to make reparation. So often, though, these feelings are destructive. Indeed, Bradshaw (1988) coined the striking phrase 'toxic shame' to describe their damaging effect. Such shame will look for the punishment it feels it deserves.

How does this come about? Always it is fostered in significant relationships, most fundamentally the family, but also in school, religious upbringing and cultural pressures. It is normal for parents to correct their children, but at the same time the love they give reassures their child that she is secure and cared for. Freud described the messages the child receives and internalises as the superego. If, however, parents are excessively strict, punishing their child frequently, angrily critical of her lapses from perfection, and giving only conditional love, then when she introjects or takes these experiences into her psyche, an inner Critic is created, who tells her that she is defective in herself. Soon, even when her parents are absent, she criticises and shames herself – 'bad girl!' 'you're stupid!' 'you're no good!' – whenever she has made some mistake. These introjects, in a more sophisticated form, stay around into adolescence and adulthood. Bad experiences at an authoritarian school or destructively competitive workplace only strengthen their hold.

Such themes come home to roost in the dying – they may see their impending death as their ultimate failure. Their body must be defective – it has cancer. But often, behind this negative interpretation, lies a lifetime of shame and guilt. Their stories are many. Typical examples might be:

- He was always compared unfavourably with his elder brother by their parents.
- She felt it was her fault when her alcoholic mother died of cirrhosis of the liver.
- A drunk driver, he killed a mother and her daughter on a pedestrian crossing.
- She had an abortion as a teenager.
- He has been estranged from his children for ten years.
- Her mother never showed her any affection and put her in an orphanage.
- He was physically abused as a child by his violent father.
- A devout Catholic, in her teens she had an illegitimate child adopted.
- His parents were critical of his poor academic performance; his school did not notice that he was dyslexic.

As a way of protecting themselves, people who experience inappropriate guilt or shame may either conceal their stories or they may develop psychological defences to reduce their distress: denial, dissociation from feelings, alcoholism, eating disorders, self-harm, compulsive caring and workaholism are examples.

In essence, toxic guilt or shame is healed by self-acceptance. This, however, is easier said than done. Life scripts are deeply imprinted and not readily changed. Fundamental to helping the patient is for her to be able to speak honestly about her shame or guilt in a climate of acceptance and care. It is only when their true origins are revealed that change can take place. Bradshaw (1988) calls this process externalisation:

- This means the patient may need to talk not only with staff but also with others who have some connection with his memories, particularly family, and who can be supportive to him.

- In dealing with shame and guilt, it is particularly important that we clinicians listen empathically and without judgement, whatever our personal views may be about what the patient is telling us.

- People in the grip of shame will tend to invalidate their experience. Irrationally, they may feel it is their fault that their father beat them frequently, or that their mother abandoned them. Their experience needs, therefore, to be legitimised, that is that they did not deserve their mistreatment and they are justified in the anger they feel at this abuse.

- Shamed people need to know that they are acceptable just as they are; they do not have to be 'perfect'.

- Some people find that a religious ritual of forgiveness is helpful to them, especially if they have *genuinely* contravened their own values. The minister has an important role here – he or she is a mediator between the patient and her God, their ultimate source of forgiveness and acceptance. In this context, forgiveness may be either about the patient forgiving herself for some misdemeanour, or forgiving another person who has wronged her. One woman would not allow her family to visit her or be given information about her illness, though they would come to the ward every day. It was only on the day she died that she allowed them to look around the curtains surrounding her bed. She never said why she behaved as she did, but it was clear she found it unbearable to be seen by them – a hallmark of shame. That final, conditional, meeting was at least a gesture towards reconciliation, towards a healing of her alienation.

GRIEF

The dying, and their loved ones, are no strangers to grief. It touches them in many ways:

- The dying person may have been recently bereaved of a family member.

- There may be unresolved past losses such as of a son or daughter dying in childhood.

- Anticipatory grieving – the dying person grieves for the family he will lose when he dies; his family begins to grieve for him as his health steadily deteriorates. Sometimes, with slowly progressive illnesses such as dementia, family members may slowly distance themselves over months or longer from someone they feel is no longer the person they knew. In a sense, he has become dead to them while his body still lives.

- Social losses – of status, money and work.

- Bodily losses – losing a leg, a breast, an eye or any other body part. Furthermore, individual organs will connote losses related to their *raison d'être*. Thus, a mastectomy may result in feelings of loss of sexual attractiveness.

- Loss of function – becoming, for example, paraplegic, blind or incontinent.

In one study, 17 per cent of patients referred to psychiatric out-patients had unresolved grief reactions (Worden 2003, p.1). Complicated grief, then, is a potent source of chronic psychological symptoms. Queen Victoria, who remained in mourning for 40 years after her beloved husband, Prince Albert, died of typhus, is a famous example.

Parkes (Worden 2003, p.26) describes four phases of mourning. The first phase is of numbness, an initial psychic protection against the unbearable pain of the loss. This is followed by a second phase of yearning, when the bereaved person pines for the return of the loved one and feels angry at her for not coming back. In the third phase, the mourner experiences despair and finds it difficult to function in everyday life, becoming disorganised. In the fourth and final phase, that of reorganisation, he begins to put his life back together again.

Grieving can present with a huge number of manifestations, such as:

- *Feelings*: sadness, anger, guilt, anxiety, loneliness, numbness.

- *Body sensations*: tight chest, depersonalisation, breathlessness, tiredness.

- *Thinking*: disbelief, confusion, preoccupation, hallucinations of the dead person.

- *Behaviour*: crying, sleep disturbance, social withdrawal, sighing.

Darwin (1872) observed that animals such as monkeys grieve. Does human crying, then, relate to mammalian distress calls when individuals are lost and separated from their group, particularly in the case of young animals (Shapiro and Forrest 2004, p.93)? Human parents find it very difficult to ignore their baby crying. Their natural instinct is to pick her up, comfort her and reassure her that she is not alone. It is no wonder that tearfulness is such a part of grief – it is the body keening for the lost loved one.

There are particular problems in providing counselling support for grief in the dying, notably the short time scale. Mourning may take one or two years to complete; it is hardly going to resolve in someone with only a few weeks to live, especially if it is a complicated grief reaction. Having said that, I have seen many elderly, dying people who take to their beds, wanting to die so that they can rejoin their loved one in the after-life. They become very quiet as if they feel hopeful that their separation will soon be ended. For others, the intensity of their feelings may be blunted by tranquillising medication they take for other reasons.

Although, then, Worden (2003) talks about the four tasks of mourning – to accept the reality of the loss, to work through the pain of grief, to adjust to the permanent absence of the deceased, and to relocate emotions invested in the deceased back into life – most of this will simply not be possible in those close to dying. So, what is to be done?

Grieving people usually do take comfort in talking about their loss. Listening empathically may, therefore, be all that is needed. They may wish to talk through some unresolved issue such as guilt. They may wish to reminisce about past times with the deceased. They may prefer not to talk. So, rather than the big agendas of long-term mourning, this is about sensing what the dying person needs in relation to grief support right now. Attend to what her psyche presents, not what you feel it ought to present in order to follow a theoretical model. This is triage work. The individual's unconscious knows what mourning needs to be carried out in the few weeks left in that person's life and what can simply be held. There may be unexpected results. One story on this theme has always moved me. It concerned one of the animal keepers at a zoo who was admitted, terminally ill, to a palliative care unit. A new baby elephant had been born at the zoo and she wished very much that she could see it but she was too ill to return there. We see here the loss she was experiencing of her place of work. Since she couldn't move, they decided to bring the baby elephant to her at the hospice. She was wheeled, in her bed, outside the building where she met the new arrival. I imagine that meeting and then saying goodbye

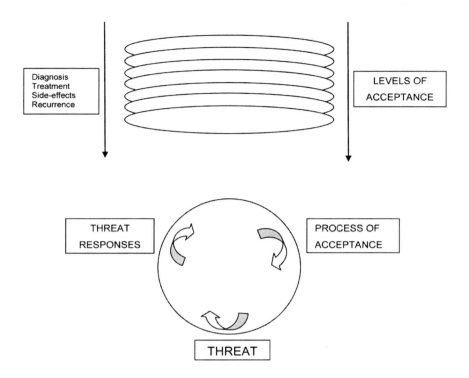

Figure 7.1 Spiral of acceptance of dying

to the elephant was also a way for her to say goodbye to the zoo, a ritual of letting go more powerful than words alone.

While I have been talking about professional help, patients also receive considerable support from other patients. They may well find it easier to talk to each other than to staff. The sad corollary of this is that they may also grieve when their new friend dies and it then becomes the task of their clinicians to support them in yet another loss.

THE SPIRAL OF ACCEPTANCE

In a famous study, the Swiss psychiatrist Elisabeth Kübler-Ross (1969) described a sequence of stages that the dying go through – denial and isolation, anger, bargaining, depression, acceptance – in their journey towards death. Unfortunately, reality is less tidy than this neat linear sequence. Just about any emotion, including feelings she did not list, can surface at any time during the dying process. And yet it is true that the mortally ill do tend to move towards acceptance. It may be more helpful to imagine this process as spiral, rather than linear.

Figure 7.1 illustrates a hypothesis for explaining the apparently random variations of feelings in the dying process. There are multiple layers to acceptance. A patient may have gone through the process of acceptance at one level, such as the diagnosis, only to be confronted by a new threat, such as recurrence of the cancer, which re-evokes the threat feelings – fear, anger, depression, sadness. In the dying, multiple threats may pile on top of each other so fast that it may feel as though there is not enough time to process them all. They are at different stages of acceptance for each of the different crises they encounter. Furthermore, the threats faced may bring to the surface old unhealed memories with their attendant feelings. Some patients, for example, who had developed the same cancer as one of their parents told me of their fears of dying in agony which is how they perceived their parent's death.

And yet, some do reach a deep acceptance of their dying, calm and silent at their ending, not even needing any medications. My experience of being in their room with such people, which other hospice workers I have talked to vouch for, is not so much one of sorrow or distress but rather of peacefulness. Here is a description of a Buddhist woman's death:

> Harriet's favourite Ngöndro chants…played softly over and over. A great peace had settled on the room… Friends came in without speaking, sat in silence, and left. Sometimes the nurses would come to stand by the bed and whisper a prayer… Harriet's breathing had changed. I knelt by the bed and placed my mala [rosary]…in her hand. The whole room felt so sacred that my feeble attempt at…'prayer' seemed…almost irreverent. I united my breathing with hers. In a timeless space beyond sorrow or pain, thoughts rose and subsided… Then the sun came out to shine through the crystal that stirred in a light breeze, to spread dancing shapes of rainbow light around Harriet's head on the pillow. It took care of itself, in the silence of indescribable peace. She gave three long gentle outbreaths. Her last outbreath coincided exactly with the last long deep syllable, and the chanting ceased (Cornish 1994, p.18).

CHAPTER 8

Euthanasia

DEFINITIONS
Euthanasia

The literal meaning of euthanasia, coming from the Greek words *eu* and *thanatos*, is 'good death'. Nowadays, euthanasia has a more specific meaning – the intentional killing of one person by another, usually to relieve suffering.

Voluntary and involuntary euthanasia

'Voluntary euthanasia' implies one person voluntarily asking another to end her life to relieve distress. 'Involuntary euthanasia' is where a person is unable to indicate his wishes because of, for example, dementia or unconsciousness, or because he is a newborn, and a decision is taken on his behalf by another. It is also used when a doctor takes steps to end another person's life without consulting her, even if that person is able to communicate her wishes.

Active and passive euthanasia

'Active euthanasia' means one person actively carrying out euthanasia on another person, for example by lethal injection. 'Passive euthanasia' is a term used to mean letting a person die through discontinuation of treatment that is not curing the disease, or simply letting nature take its course in the case of a terminal illness.

Assisted suicide

This is where one person, usually a doctor, provides the means for another, who is terminally ill, to take his own life. Examples include provision of a lethal dose of drugs, either as tablets or by setting up an intravenous infusion which the terminally ill person can activate himself.

Living wills (advance directives)

These are written declarations about the patient's wishes concerning treatment, usually for a terminal illness. In this he can set out what treatment he *doesn't* want, but he cannot insist on having a particular treatment – this is a medical decision. He may appoint a proxy to speak for him if he is unable to do so. These documents are legally valid and so their stipulations must be respected. In fact, even a verbal statement alone by the patient as to his wishes carries the same force. The Terrence Higgins Trust (see the Resources section at the end of this book) provides blank wills.

THE LAW ON EUTHANASIA

Voluntary, involuntary and active euthanasia, and assisted suicide, are illegal in Great Britain. Euthanasia is illegal in most countries. There are exceptions, such as Holland, Belgium, Switzerland and the state of Oregon in the USA.

When a person is terminally ill, such as with an advanced cancer that is no longer responding to curative treatment, it is certainly permissible legally and ethically to stop treatments that are no longer working but simply drawing out the process of dying. In the same way, it is regarded as acceptable practice in the United Kingdom to give treatments such as pain-relieving drugs to decrease suffering even when a possible secondary, but not intended, effect of this might be to shorten life. This is the ethical principle of double effect, which, however, proponents of euthanasia do not regard as valid. In practice, medications such as morphine can be used safely to control pain and many patients take this drug for months or longer – clearly their life is not being shortened.

There have been repeated unsuccessful attempts to pass a bill through Parliament legalising euthanasia in some form.

SOCIETY

Opinion polls from the general public have shown a majority to be in favour of euthanasia. Polls taken from doctors usually show the opposite. Palliative care organisations in the UK are against euthanasia. My impression is that the great majority of individuals working in palliative care are similarly opposed.

ETHICS

Euthanasia has been a hotly debated ethical issue for decades. It is beyond the scope of this book to provide a detailed critique of the arguments involved. In summary, ethical principles invoked both for and against euthanasia include:

- *The sanctity of life*: this holds that life is sacred and inviolate.

- *Autonomy*: everyone has the right to make their own choices, including whether to end their life.

- *Duty of care*: patients have a right to be cared for competently.

- *Double effect*: this states that it is permissible to give a treatment for one reason which *may* have as a secondary but unintended consequence, the effect of shortening a patient's life.

- *Beneficence*: actions taken should be in the best interests of the patient.

- *Non-maleficence*: do not cause harm.

From these apparently simple statements has been spun a vast web of impassioned debate. Everyone reading this book will have a view, and if it is that you are neutral, then that in itself is a view. While I personally am opposed to euthanasia, I do have considerable sympathy for the feelings of patients who broach the subject. The life instinct is very powerful. For a patient to wish to end her life is a sign that she feels all hope is gone, an indicator of crisis.

How can we, as clinicians, respond constructively to this? It doesn't matter what your viewpoint is, it is the same practical question. If you are against euthanasia, you wouldn't consider it anyway. If you are for euthanasia, it is illegal. So, either way, we need to look for other ways of supporting patients in their plight. One way to do this is to work from their motivations. These may include one or more of the following:

- fear of unbearable suffering
- fear of prolonged suffering
- loss of control
- depressive illness
- spiritual distress
- a considered choice made in advance of the terminal illness
- the fall-back position
- on and off
- family pressures.

RESPONSES
Fear of unbearable suffering

Many patients fear that as the cancer progresses their suffering, particularly their pain, will exponentially increase until it becomes an unbearable, living hell. They may cite stories of relatives whom they saw die in agony. Here, they need to know that symptom control in general and pain control in particular is highly successful in relieving suffering. They can find this hard to believe since they may have been in inadequately treated pain for months on end. In this case, the proof of the pudding is in the eating. They need to experience the effects of effective symptom control.

A woman was admitted to a hospice where I was working, with kidney cancer and bone metastases. She had had severe unrelieved back pain on and off for years. In hospital she had requested extra painkillers. The staff thought she was addicted and they wouldn't give her any more. The truth was she was desperate – her pain was so severe. One night she decided to cut her wrists. She was found in the morning in a pool of blood but still alive. When she came to the hospice, her pain was relatively simple to treat with morphine and non-steroidal anti-inflammatory drugs. I remember asking her a fortnight later – she was free of pain by then – did she still feel suicidal? Her answer was no.

It may, of course, have been true that a relative died in pain, but this would have been from a lack of expertise on the part of the doctor treating their relative, not that the pain was untreatable. It is worth exploring, too, the patient's perception of the death of his loved one. Sometimes, patients' own distress may colour how they view what happened. Enquiry may reveal an assumption of suffering even if the relative did not show signs of distress. Equally, if it is clear that the death was agonising, patients need to know that you have heard them and empathise with their anguish and even outrage at what happened – and that you will make sure that they do not suffer in the same way.

Fear of prolonged suffering

This is more about the length of suffering than its intensity – the thought that an illness will drag on for months or years with no end in sight. It is Macbeth's plaint on being told that his queen is dead: 'Tomorrow, and tomorrow, and tomorrow, / Creeps in this petty pace from day to day, / To the last syllable of recorded time...' (Shakespeare 1905, p.867). Ask the patient how long he thinks he has to live. I have often encountered the situation where he says a year or two, whereas I can see that it is more likely to be a week or two. This is one of the few situations where it can be helpful to tell a patient he hasn't got long to live. He may actually feel deeply relieved; it won't be long before he dies. He can manage that.

However, some, such as those with motor neurone disease (MND), may be significantly incapacitated and may actually have years to live. This is highlighted by the story of Diane Pretty who sought a legal ruling that her husband could assist her suicide because she had advanced MND. Her case was eventually dismissed by the European Court of Human Rights and she died in a hospice in 2002. Other individuals, however, despite severe progressive disability, wish to continue living. The physicist Stephen Hawking, who has had MND for 44 years, is an example. What makes the difference? Each story is unique, but one common denominator is the sense of meaning. We have already considered Victor Frankl's experiences in a concentration camp and his observation that it was those inmates with a sense of meaning in their lives who were most likely to survive (Frankl 2004). Perhaps in an analogous way the attitude of those with long-term fatal illnesses to euthanasia depends crucially on whether they see any meaning to their life, any reason to continue their existence. It is in the end a question of individual perception which reflects that person's unique make-up and history. It is also an existential choice.

There is no point in pretending that, for some, the experience of going through such illnesses won't generate considerable distress. It is all the more important to ask, then, what can in practice be helpful? For a start, such patients need to know that they are cared for. This may seem self-evident, but, so often, they have had bad experiences of not being well looked after in hospital, of their time-consuming needs being ignored on a busy, understaffed, acute medical ward. They need to know, then, that the hospice staff will give them the necessary time, day in, day out, whether this be nursing, medical, counselling or pastoral; the theme of 'watch with me' again. And this sums up the steadfast commitment needed in the care of such patients. Also, look out for what *can* make their life meaningful for them. Listen to and respect their story and point of view. It may be worth exploring with them, if they wish to, how they came to their belief. See if there is anything they *would* like to do. This may be something as simple as having visits home or a chance, if they are well enough, to go out for a drive in the country. This needs to come from them; well-meaning suggestions of what others think they ought to like will not help. Is this approach useful? Although I don't wish to deny the difficulties of supporting these patients in their suffering, in practice my experience has been that they are not *of necessity* in a fixed state of hopelessness; it is possible for there to be good days as well as bad days.

It is also important to find out if they want treatment, such as antibiotics for pneumonia. It may seem obvious that they would not, but in practice I have been surprised by how often they will decide to have the treatment 'on this occasion'. Many, however, are clear that they do not want any further treatment, which is their right, and the ward staff need to know this and to record this information in the clinical notes. Some patients make a Living Will to confirm their decision in writing.

Loss of control

Similar considerations apply to loss of control, which comes in many forms in the dying: paraplegia, incontinence, confusion, loss of speech, weakness, blindness. The list is long. These losses can evoke deep fear. There may be a feeling of regressing to childhood, even having to wear nappies again. Patients may feel shamed or they may rage at their incapacity. I have come across patients with MND who, unable to move or speak, have resorted to wailing as their only way of communicating their distress. People in such crisis situations may request euthanasia. As ever, it is important to look below the surface. Let us return to the experience of very young babies. They are helpless and depend on their mother to provide for their needs. But the consequences of deprivation of these needs may be very serious. As Winnicott (1988, p.86) puts it:

> Behind these needs…babies are liable to the most severe anxieties that can be imagined. If left for too long (hours, minutes) without familiar and human contact they have experiences which we can only describe by such words as: going to pieces; falling for ever; dying and dying and dying; losing all vestige of hope of the renewal of contacts.

It is not surprising that such elemental experiences may be re-evoked in some people when they are plunged into a re-living of their newborn helplessness. No wonder they wish to escape this anguish. In supporting them, we return again to the crucial importance of the nursing care provided: warmth, touch, massage, feeding, washing, a quiet voice. All of these resonate with the patient's earliest experiences in life, and, if this was seriously deprived, they provide a counterbalance, a good experience of being cared for, that helps to meet and calm their primal terror.

Some, however, live this experience differently. Marie de Hennezel (1997) tells the moving story of Danièle, a young woman with amyotrophic lateral sclerosis, a form of MND which had rendered her paralysed and unable to speak. She could only communicate by blinking her eyelids and by pressing with a finger on the lever of a word processor to form words slowly and with difficulty on the screen. She described how one day she could no longer hold her psychological anguish at bay.

> I've never gone through anything remotely like that: Screams were coming out of my chest, loud, raucous, uncontrollable screams, and I thought, The children will hear. And *IT* kept screaming. My whole body shook and fought against the paralysis. (p.103)

And yet she was also able to write to her sister: 'but I feel in very good health! Everything is working fine – except for my outer layer!' (p.93). She reflected: 'I created my illness as a response to being abandoned. Cunning! But now I have proof that people love me, and I want to live, but my virus won't listen' (p.92). Virus was the name she gave her illness. She commented about her decision to take up the challenge of her illness: 'I can tell you my weapons: Avoid all comparisons with the past and learn to live this as a particularly long and difficult passage' (p.121). She had a dream in which she and others are in a field of land mines. 'Some people step on the mines, others stand still to avoid stepping on them and I say to myself, Doing nothing so as to avoid dying is not a life! So I go forward aware of the risk.' Saddened when her sister leaves for Cuba, she listened to Fauré's *Requiem* 'about which she had once said, "If there's one piece of music that leads you to God, it's this"' (p.148). She professed no belief in God. Just before her death, she wrote: 'Happiness comes unannounced even on the wings of illness' (p.164).

Depressive illness

Suicidal feelings, as already discussed, may be a symptom of a depressive illness. This obviously needs assessment and treatment, and has been considered in Chapter 7. It is not enough to assume if someone terminally ill feels depressed and want to die, there is nothing that can be done. That way, they will miss out on treatment that can relieve their suffering, including their self-destructive feelings.

Spiritual distress

This may mimic clinical depression and is considered in Chapter 10. Here, the feeling of wanting to die emanates from an archetypal level of the psyche, a level which communicates in metaphors. Dying, in this case, may symbolise the transition from one state of being to the next; the former state passes away. An example is the transition from adolescence to adulthood; in traditional societies, rites of passage for this journey include a symbol such as circumcision or other wounding to express the loss, the little death. It misses the mark to take this 'dying' literally. Many teenagers do and there is a high suicide rate in adolescence. The same applies for existential crises in those with advanced cancer. These may be *not only* about facing actual death but also about leaving behind a former way of life that no longer serves the dying person; she may then find that her past behaviour, such as heavy drinking or workaholism, masked an emptiness in her life which is now revealed. It would, equally, be a mistake for the clinician to take a request for euthanasia from such a patient at the literal level. His task, rather, is about helping the patient with her inner spiritual transition.

A considered choice made in advance of the terminal illness

Some people will have thought carefully about having a terminal or a chronic, progressive illness and have decided they would prefer to end their life rather than go through the suffering entailed. They may commit suicide. They may secretly seek euthanasia or assisted suicide with the help of a friend, relative or a doctor in agreement with their view. Some may consider going to Switzerland to obtain euthanasia. Some may simply draw up a Living Will to ensure they are not given life-preserving treatments such as antibiotics when they are dying. These last are the ones most likely to be encountered in a palliative care setting. It can sometimes be worth exploring with them, if they so wish, what it was that was unacceptable beneath their rational consideration. 'Unacceptable' means 'I don't want it', and that implies, inevitably, feelings about what they imagine their illness will bring, such as suffering or loss of control. It may be that some of their feelings are based on factual inaccuracies such as that pain cannot be controlled – these, at least, can be dispelled.

Another problem is trying to predict what will happen. No living will can legislate for all eventualities and real life often brings the unexpected in terms of progression of a terminal illness. Equally, the patient may change her mind when she finds that the experience of a particular medical complication is bearable and she would like to have treatment for it. So, the key is to ask the patient at the time of the clinical crisis what her wishes are concerning further treatment. Ensure this is recorded in her notes if it differs from her Living Will.

The fall-back position

Some people talk about euthanasia in a different sense. They are for it and would want it if it were available, indeed they may even have considered going abroad for euthanasia – but not just yet. It is like a fall-back position that they might return to if needed.

On and off

There are patients who fluctuate from day to day. On bad days when they feel upset or are in pain, they wish they were dead, but on good days they feel that they want to go on living. Clearly it is their distress that needs attention, whether through symptom control or counselling.

Family pressures

Families may want to support patients in their request for euthanasia. They may, too, speak out when the patient is unable to do so. This often happens close to the patient's death. 'Please put him out of his misery, doctor,' is a frequent comment, as is: 'You wouldn't treat a dog like that.' Often, the patient is actually comfortable and asleep, and these comments reflect the family's understandable distress at seeing their loved one so changed – skeletally thin, pale, unconscious, catheterised, bandaged. It is indeed deeply upsetting to see someone you love come to such a pass, but it is important for the staff attending the patient to demonstrate to the family that he isn't suffering and that any pain will be immediately treated.

There are patients requesting euthanasia who do so because they feel guilty at the slowness of their dying, which they feel is upsetting their family. So often, the family, by contrast, is deeply committed to accompanying them during his final illness and are hurt that they should think such a thing. The clinician's job here is to ensure that both sides are talking to each other – they may not have done so for fear of causing distress.

Communication may have broken down between the patient and her family and this may be reflected in a despairing request for euthanasia. Here again, the care provided is key to offering the patient a way out of her isolation and back into human contact. Sometimes, it may be possible to work with the patient and family together towards healing their rift.

Other darker family motives may occasionally surface. Evidence submitted to the House of Lords Select Committee on Medical Ethics which reported on euthanasia (House of Lords 1994) included a case where a family tried to persuade hospice doctors to give escalating doses of analgesia to their dying relative. It later came to light that they stood to gain £20,000 if he died before a certain date.

CHAPTER 9

Family Matters

FAMILY SYSTEMS

A useful way to view family relationships is to think of the family as a system in which each member interacts with the others as do parts of the body with the whole (Satir 1972). The psychological health of each individual depends, then, not only on his own psyche but also on his relationships with the other family members. When problems arise in a family, this is then seen as an effect of the interactions in the family system, rather than as the fault of an individual. This is like the idea that an individual has many intrapsychic subpersonalities. This approach was developed from systems theory which explains the nature of complex systems in the natural world, science and human groups. An important element of this is homeostasis, whereby the system (the family) maintains stability through the dynamic relationships of the parts (the individuals). In families this may be healthy or dysfunctional; either way it will tend to be self-perpetuating.

An important way of getting a sense of the individual family system is to draw a family tree, as shown in Figure 9.1. This is far better than a list of names because it immediately gives a picture of the geography of the family. Doing a family tree with the patient may reveal much information, or highlight areas the patient would rather not talk about, which itself is a form of information. Questions suggest themselves. How did Ricky die at the age of three? What effect has it had on the family? Are Jane and Alan still in contact after their divorce? What effect did this have on Tara? How does the family view Jane's new lesbian relationship with Dee? Are Sarah and Jane worried about the family history of breast cancer?

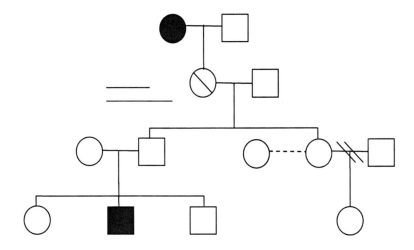

Key: —married --- cohabiting □ male ■ died ○ female ⊘ patient
    \\ divorced

Figure 9.1 Example of family tree (fictional)

Family roles

Members of the family will tend to assume different roles. As a central player, the patient will be assigned the sick role, although some will fight against this and try to live their usual lives, going to work, driving and so on. Sometimes, it is the spouses who have been in the sick role for many years and they may find it difficult to relinquish their status. From time to time I have seen partners who are upset and angry that their partner, who has taken care of them for years, is now dying and unable to support them. 'What about me?' they ask plaintively, struggling with the responsibility of living their own lives; or they may not believe that the dying person can no longer look after them. And the patient may struggle to continue her accustomed, self-perpetuating caring role, despite her own weakness and need of support.

Another role is that of the spokesperson. This is not necessarily the partner of the patient. Some who assume this role may privately lack confidence in their ability and compensate with overconfidence and even aggression. There may be competition for this position and rivals may talk to staff separately, with the risk that staff become caught up in the family conflicts. The spokesperson may think it his role to take over responsibility for decisions which the patient is competent to make herself. It is therefore important to keep referring to the patient and asking if she is in agreement with plans under discussion.

Other roles include the scapegoat, the clown, the carer, the rebel, the pleaser, and so on. Though these roles may relate to an individual's character, they don't define the totality of that person. Curiously, if a family member dies or moves away, his role may be adopted by another relative. It is a well-known and tragic cliché, which fortunately is less prevalent now, that, when a father died, his young son would be exhorted to become 'the man of the house'.

These patterns are more obvious in dysfunctional families. One member of the family may express repressed conflictual energies for the whole clan, and will be labelled as difficult or rebellious. She is being scapegoated for the others' denied shadow. The Indian film *Monsoon Wedding* portrayed this clearly – in it, a young woman tried to tell her family that her much respected uncle had sexually abused her when she was a girl, but her family's reaction was of anger at her for making such accusations followed by an attempt to ignore them.

Families may split into camps; individuals may not talk to each other, or break off all contact. Nevertheless, they may find themselves looking at each other across the bed of their dying relative. Some can't even bear to do this and will stagger their visits so that they do not encounter their family enemy. Ward staff may need to mediate between the hostile camps in the making of such decisions.

Families are the crucible for the sometimes byzantine workings of the Oedipus complex, which Freud described using the myth of Oedipus who, unwittingly, killed his father and married his mother (Jacobs 1998). It is a normal stage of development during which the child wishes to possess the parent of the opposite sex and eliminate the parent of the same sex. This matrix can be generalised to any triangular relationship at any age; typically, two will form an alliance and exclude the third. The bigger the family, the greater the number of such triangles that may be formed. Thus, one bereaved man told me how he had had a perfect childhood. His father favoured his brother while his mother favoured him. What he left out was how his father routinely condemned and ignored him but indulged his brother.

The various roles that family members adopt suggest a theatrical analogy. It is as though they are in a play with a plot, a family script, in which each player performs his predetermined part rigidly, and the self-destructive family stories repeat themselves endlessly. The enmity of the Montagues and Capulets in Shakespeare's *Romeo and Juliet* is an example. Family therapists help families to change these scripts and explore new more constructive ones. This is long-term work and so beyond the scope of the time-limited hospice scenario. However, it may be possible to work with an individual on moving out of his habitual stuck role in the family. This may not be easy as other members of the family will often try, albeit unconsciously, to prevent this change.

Family meetings

Families interact in bewilderingly complex ways with staff. Any family member might talk informally with any member of staff at any time. However, there are times when more formal meetings with families are arranged. Many topics may be covered, so involvement by the doctor, nurse and social worker together may be needed, and the conversation may slide between medical, nursing and psychosocial issues.

One of the most emotive issues is about a patient going home. Most hospice beds are for short stays and family reactions to the idea of the patient going home vary from enthusiastic to hostile. This is not necessarily related to the physical capability of the patient or her relatives; it is more attitudinal. I can recall one patient whose partner cared for him at home despite the fact that he was almost completely paralysed, and needing total nursing care and intermittent use of a ventilator; she was determined to do it. Another patient was ambulant and able to take care of himself, but suffered from disabling anxiety and an attendant host of psychosomatic symptoms for which he was admitted to the hospice. New symptoms would appear when discharge was mentioned and his partner was insistent on him staying until these were addressed.

Points to remember in family meetings include the following:

- It is inevitable that different meetings may have different members of the family attending, expressing different views. Information from a previous meeting may have to be repeated for new attenders and agreements renegotiated.

- Make sure you know the names and relationships of all those present. Asking for this information helps to break the ice.

- Even if one person is dominating the conversation, try to keep aware of what's happening with the other family members – are they restless, seemingly uninterested, shaking their heads vehemently in disagreement or supportive? At an appropriate moment, you can then include them: 'I noticed that you were looking a bit worried when Andrew was talking of going home'.

- Where feasible, work with the family dynamics. Build on the strengths that they have, the ways they cooperate with each other in supporting the patient and each other.

- Where there is disagreement between family members, it may not be possible to do in-depth counselling work, but it is still important to look for ways of mediating cooperation, a pragmatic approach akin to the resolution of political disputes. Fisher, Ury and Patton (1992), in their book *Getting to Yes*, set out the essentials of such negotiations, based on their experience of international politics. They stress, first, the importance of keeping the people and the problem distinct. So often, the two become intertwined and blame flies back and forth – the patient blames his wife because he insists on going home tomorrow and she won't have it, while she blames him for not accepting that she has bad angina and so could not provide the nursing care needed. Second, focus on interests rather than positions; interests are the 'wants' behind the stances taken. He wants to go home; she doesn't want another heart attack. Third, following on from this, create choices that are to the participants' *mutual* advantage: perhaps he could go home at weekends when other members of the family are available; perhaps he could have an outing home during the week with a nurse accompanying him; perhaps nursing support at home could be arranged; and so on. Fourth, use objective criteria that all can agree to in making decisions: an example would be the likelihood of response to chemotherapy when deciding whether to have this treatment.

- Make sure that, before the end of the meeting you check with those who haven't spoken as to whether they wish to say anything. This is particularly important with children, who may have been relegated to the background as if they were

invisible but who may still be listening intently to what is
being said.

- The members of the clinical team taking part in the meeting
  are, in the way they work together, implicitly modelling
  cooperation and good communication to the family – rather
  than conflict and splitting.

- Arrange a further meeting if necessary.

- It can sometimes help to provide a written summary of the
  points discussed in the meeting, particularly if the family are
  distressed and so finding it hard to recall the details of what
  was agreed.

What stories are there in Althea's family? Winston confides in Maureen,
the night sister:

Althea

Althea is less well now having had an episode of confusion because
of high blood calcium levels. Winston visits in the evenings because
of his work. While she dozes he takes a break. Maureen finds him
alone in the sitting room watching a film on television. He is clearly
worried. As they talk, he tells her that he had an affair a year before
Althea developed breast cancer. She was very upset, though she
forgave him. He wonders if this crisis might have brought on her
illness. He talks, too, of her parents who have never really accepted
him – there are tensions at home when they are looking after the
children. He thinks it is because of his colour, though Althea resists
this idea.

Apart from the therapeutic value to Winston of talking about his concerns,
the information gleaned may be important in any future discussions
involving him, Althea and her parents. Gradually, over time, further talks
with Althea and her family will build up a jigsaw of information, a piecing
together of the family story.

TALKING TO CHILDREN

Many years ago, I had a conversation with a man in his thirties. When he
was ten his father died. His family didn't tell him; instead they said that his
father had gone on a long holiday and would be back soon. He waited

impatiently and longingly. A year later, he discovered the truth. He was furious – and was still furious over 20 years later. He had been excluded from one of the most significant events in his life and he had been deceived by his own mother.

Families, understandably, want to spare children pain if their parent is dying. So often, children are sent off to play when I talk with patients and their families; or they are kept away. 'Have you talked with your children about what is happening?' I enquire. 'Well no. We've just said that Mum's not very well and needs to be in hospital.' Silently, I feel a concern. As the example above illustrates, children do need to be involved and prepared; they are worse off if they are not, and they have to live with the consequences of an unacknowledged grief.

Counselling children needs specialist skills. Social workers with training in working psychologically with families and children, come to the fore here. However, in hospices, any member of the clinical team may be involved and there are some general points to bear in mind. I don't have much experience of talking with children dying of cancer, so I have not included this topic here. The reader is referred to other texts (Bluebond-Langner 1978).

Levels of understanding increase gradually with age, as any parent knows. Very young children live in the present and it is only gradually that the concept of time develops. A three-year-old is primarily concerned that Mummy is here now and the idea that she may not be here in six months' time is beyond her grasp. A ten-year-old will, however, more readily understand the idea of something happening in the future and will need preparation accordingly.

Similarly, the idea of death develops gradually, as is shown in Table 9.1. Young children love peek-a-boo games where something disappears and returns, but the concept that a loved one will *never* return comes slowly. When my wife and I took our young children to see the Disney cartoon *Bambi*, our three-year-old daughter watched the scene where Bambi's mother is killed by the hunter, leaving the the fawn wandering in the forest orphaned, and then asked several times with increasing urgency and anxiety, 'But where's the mummy?' She understood and felt anxiety at the separation but did not grasp the concept of the permanence of death. As children grow older, they slowly gain experience from their surroundings about death – they may have seen pets or other animals die or they may

Table 9.1 Development of understanding of death by children. (adapted from Herbert 1996, pp.19–24). Ages given are approximate

AGE	CONCEPTUALISATION OF DEATH
A few weeks	Separation anxiety
6–8 months	Attachment to parents
3 years	Aware of death but understanding very limited
4 years	Yearning for absent parents and awaits their return
5 years	Separation from dead parent understood
5 years	Dead people cannot move
6 years	Death is irrevocable
6 years	Death has a physical cause and is not the child's fault
6 years	Cessation of bodily function
7 years	Death is universal
8 years	The dead person cannot feel anything
8–9 years	A child knows he can die himself
12 years	The appearance of a dead person is understood

have thought about leaves dying, a dead tree or a ruined building and gained understanding accordingly. Television is a major source of information, both realistic and unrealistic, as are books. Children will, of course, talk to each other and here, too, fact and fantasy mingle.

The same applies to concepts of illness. Young children may understand illness in terms of words they have heard such as 'poorly' or 'not well' or they may use illnesses they have encountered as references: Granny had bronchitis; a friend broke her arm; her brother had appendicitis. A fifteen-year-old will understand the idea that the body is made up of cells and cancer starts as a cell that continues to multiply without stopping, but this would not be an appropriate explanation for a five-year-old.

To make matters more complicated, children of the same age will have different levels of understanding; guides to childhood development are only approximate. Further, emotional maturation does not always keep pace with intellectual understanding. A child may understand mentally that his father is dying but he may find this knowledge unbearably painful and shut down his feelings by dissociating or becoming depressed or having tantrums. Children with a parent or sibling who has had a long-term illness may be more likely to have a more sophisticated understanding of illness and its attendant emotional fall-out. Normally, the people best placed to assess an individual child's level of development are the parents. So, any discussion with children needs to be in close cooperation with them.

These factors were movingly demonstrated in the film *Contact* based on the book by Carl Sagan. The story centres around an astronomer obsessively searching for extra-terrestrial intelligence. In a flash-back, we see her as a girl whose mother died at her birth and who shares her father's love of astronomy and short-wave radio. He dies suddenly and, at the funeral reception, she leaves the adults, goes to her room and despairingly starts to call her father on the short-wave radio. This becomes sublimated into her adult search for alien life forms.

It may be difficult for parents to take on the task of preparing their children for a forthcoming death. While they may wish to avoid hurting them, it may also be that they are trying to avoid their own distress too; talking with a child will put them in touch with their own inner Child, who is also vulnerable and bewildered. Nevertheless, it is in the end impossible to avoid the fact of the death and it is this, more than anything, which will bring parents to speak in some fashion to their children, who do, after all, need to express their feelings and mourn just as much as adults.

Parents may take a long time exploring their feelings with the clinical staff about breaking bad news to their children, before they feel ready to do so. It may help to acknowledge their distress by saying to them: 'This must be the worst thing you have ever had to say to your children'. It can also be useful to speak about the research evidence which shows that children experience more emotional difficulties if not told. Sometimes parents find it beneficial to practise what they will say to their children with a member of staff. One woman whose husband was dying used to send her daughter to play with a neighbour every time the doctor called to prevent her being told anything. It was only when he had been in the hospice for some weeks and was close to dying that she eventually agreed, after many discussions with the clinical staff, to tell her daughter that her father was dying.

A parent may tell his child that Mummy has gone to heaven, or that she is now one of the stars in the sky, by way of explanation. Remember, in this context, that younger children will tend to take what they are told literally. If they are informed Mummy is asleep, they may fear going to sleep themselves. They will have questions: 'Why can't I go to heaven to be with Mummy?' They may even, at the funeral, want to jump into the grave to be with their loved parent. The spiritual beliefs of parents, especially concerning an after-life, will obviously influence their children's understanding. Nevertheless, any child may be curious about where Granny has gone. Children's books such as *Badger's Parting Gifts* by Susan Varley (1985) are useful in addressing this and other areas concerning dying.

Even if parents refuse to tell their children what is happening, these children will still be forming their own impressions of what is going on and, especially with the older ones, may very well be aware that their mother or father is dying. However, they don't wish to upset their parents and so say nothing – thus a game of mutual collusion develops (Bluebond-Langner 1978). They may also feel that, somehow, what has happened is their fault – a form of magical thinking. If only they had behaved better their mother would not be dying. This is another reason for talking with children – to help free them from the distress of their unnecessary self-blame. They may also make assumptions about cancer that are wrong. Some children think they can catch cancer if they eat off the plate Dad used before he died.

If they don't have an opportunity to communicate their feelings, children may instead speak through their behaviour: tantrums, nightmares and bed-wetting in the younger; truanting, shoplifting or fights in the older. When they are given the space to express themselves, children tend to move flexibly in and out of their emotions much more rapidly than adults. One moment they may be in tears and a few minutes later playing happily. Younger children may find it easier to express themselves symbolically, perhaps through their toys or an invisible friend, or through painting or clay. 'Bunny is sad', a little boy may say, holding his toy rabbit; actually, the boy is, but it eases the pain to, so to speak, put it into Bunny.

Althea

While Debbie, the social worker, is chatting with Althea, Rachel and Jack are sitting on the floor doing paintings for their mother. Soon, they bring them over. Rachel's shows Althea lying in bed. A nurse is holding a bright blue medicine bottle and Rachel, in nurse's uniform, is giving her mother the medicine. Jack has painted a superhero who is zapping green monsters with a huge ray gun. Althea has only recently had radiotherapy.

The above scenario is an opportunity for Debbie to ask the children to tell her about the paintings, as a way of beginning gently to make conscious their anxieties expressed indirectly in their paintings. This approach, play therapy, was touchingly illustrated in a wonderful book called *Dibs In Search of Self*, by Virginia Axline (1971). A child psychotherapist, she describes her therapeutic work with a small boy, Dibs, who was considered disturbed and mentally defective. Hers was a process of quiet attention while he began to come out of his shell, as he talked, played with toys and painted. She would watch as he used the sand tray, toy soldiers, dolls and animals to act out stories about his life and the traumas he had experienced. Carefully, she would comment on what was happening, letting him know he had her full attention. Slowly he blossomed and a gifted, insightful, sensitive child emerged. After the therapy finished, she met Dibs in the street and they recalled their time together: "'What did we play, Dibs?' Dibs leaned towards me. His eyes were shining. "Everything I did, you did," he whispered. "Everything I said, you said."' (p.190) – such a clear description of the therapeutic power of mirroring.

Some dying people make a memory box, which will contain memorabilia by which their children can remember them, especially in the case of the very young who may lose their conscious memory of their dead parent.

SEXUALITY AND SENSUALITY

Our present-day sentimentalised image of Cupid is of a mischievous little boy whose arrows make people fall in love. Earlier versions in Greek mythology, however, hold that, as Eros, he was the first of the gods and set the world in motion (Graves 1992). This points to a far wilder and more powerful view of this god of love. It suggests that the themes of masculinity and femininity are not just physical, but also pervade our psyches as archetypes. Jung (Storr 1998, pp.100–105) made this very point: whether we are physically male or female, our psyche is both masculine and feminine. He called the feminine aspect of the psyche in men the anima, and the masculine aspect in women the animus, these being the Latin words for soul. This complementarity is recognised in many world religions. Thus Taoism describes the T'ai Chi, the famous circle containing the intertwining principles of yin and yang, darkness and light, masculine and feminine. These polarities infuse every aspect of living: food, dance, music, art, nature as well as physical sex. It means the sensuality of eros can be expressed even where sex is not a possibility.

This is a crucial distinction in palliative care. Many people with advanced cancer are unable to have sex, but they are not excluded from eros in its wider sense. This was well expressed by one frail man who had just been admitted to a hospice and was being given his first bath in a fortnight by a nurse. As he slid luxuriously into the hot water, he said: 'This is wonderful, even better than sex.' While readers may have their own views as to the relative merits of these activities, his comment certainly emphasises the importance of the sensual.

Patients often, in the hope of eradicating a feared cancer, agree to a sexually mutilating operations. Mastectomy, orchidectomy, hysterectomy, prostatectomy: the cold clinical terms cover a deep distress at the loss of an aspect of their sexuality. They can feel a disgust at their disfigurement. Who could find them attractive now? Will their partner still love them? These considerations alone may inhibit sexual feelings, but others compound the issue:

- loss of or damage to sexual organs needed for intercourse, for example penile amputation or vulvectomy

- damage to nerve plexuses that mediate orgasm, for example radical prostatectomy or pelvic metastases

- drugs that inhibit natural sex hormones, or simply sedate

- fear by their partner of causing damage or pain during sex

- their partner feeling put off by the patient's state. This magnifies the ill person's sense of loneliness and shame

- debility – many patents are too ill even to turn over in bed let alone think about sex

- pre-existing sexual problems.

It can be seen that both internal psychological as well as external physical factors come into play. In supporting patients dealing with sexual issues, the opportunity to grieve for the loss of sexual organs, their attractiveness, and the ability to have sex with their partner, may need to be addressed. Confusingly, women who have had a mastectomy may experience the phantom presence of their nipple, just as leg amputees can still feel their absent limb. Their breast has gone, but it still makes its ghostly presence felt. It can be helpful for patients who have undergone such operations to share their feelings with their partner. A caring and supportive response may do much to restore their injured self-esteem – they are still loved despite their feelings of loss of attractiveness.

Sometimes, practical advice is helpful. One man who was catheterised, wondered if he could still have sex and was relieved to find that having a catheter need not prevent this. For those for whom sex is not possible, they may want to investigate other expressions of eros in the wider sense alluded to above. Time alone with their partner is an obvious element. Some partners like to bring food in or music that they both enjoy, or to help with the nursing care. Bringing in treasured items such as photographs from home is almost universal. If the patient is well enough, they may go out walking or for a meal. All of these may be sensual activities. Whenever I have talked to patients who have had a massage or reflexology, their response to these therapies has been one of deep pleasure and relaxation. This is open to everyone whatever their sexual situation; and there is an important message here – of valuing their physicality despite their illness and its effects on their body image. Somebody is prepared to touch them intimately even if they themselves feel self-disgust. Nurses are experts in this area. Their skill and care in giving a bath, creaming or turning a patient in bed, and changing dressings, and in how they touch the sick person can be experienced as enjoyable and comforting by the patient.

One depressed woman took advantage of a spell of good weather and spent all day outside in the garden of her hospice, protected from the sun by a parasol. She told me she would watch the clouds scudding across the blue sky and felt at peace. Her depression vanished over a fortnight. To my mind this was a sensual experience of the healing power of nature. It is interesting that traditional cultures such as in Hawaii assign genders to natural features such as rocks, streams or trees in recognition of the presence of eros in nature.

This is not a list of activities to advise. That could be imposing an external opinion on something very personal. Rather, they are examples of what individual patients have found worked for them and which they may wish to discuss with hospice staff.

Gay couples may have to contend with discrimination as well as illness. One woman told me how the hospital refused to accept that she was the partner of a patient they were treating. One doctor would repeatedly decline to give her information without checking with the patient each time. Part of the remit of my conversation with this woman was to ensure that she knew that I accepted the validity of her relationship with the patient and was ready to discuss whatever questions she had.

While there may be many difficulties, sexual desire may still make its presence felt. I recall once, on a ward round, knocking on the door of a patient's room. There was a long silence and frantic scufflings could be heard within. Eventually we were invited in and it was clear from their flushed cheeks and rapid breathing that we had unwittingly interrupted the couple in mid-coupling. After a short embarrassed conversation, we tactfully withdrew. Such nerve, was my admiring reflection as we retreated to the next patient.

PSYCHOLOGICAL TRAUMA

A number of patients I have looked after have shown signs of extreme fear bordering on terror as they realise that their cancer is inexorably advancing. They have become agitated, panicky, tearful, unable to think and experience nightmares. This is more than the usual anxiety that patients feel when facing cancer; past traumatic experiences have been re-evoked.

Palliative care patients have not infrequently had traumatic experiences. These include:

- childhood physical, emotional or sexual abuse, including extreme neglect
- childhood witnessing of such abuse

- experiencing psychological invasion: for example, refugees interrogated in prison
- experiencing or witnessing life-threatening events:
  - war memories such as of being in a concentration camp
  - cancer and its treatment
  - other illnesses: for example, the paralysis associated with MND
  - major accidents
  - physical or sexual assault.

Some may develop post-traumatic stress disorder (PTSD). Features of this (American Psychiatric Association 2000) include:

- exposure to a life-threatening event with a response that includes helplessness, horror and fear
- persistent distressing re-experiencing of the event such as through flash-backs or nightmares
- attempts to avoid triggers that recall the trauma such as people or places
- inability to recall important aspects of the event
- increased arousal such as insomnia or hypervigilance
- significant distress and impairment of functioning
- symptoms lasting more than one month.

In Chapter 7, we considered the survival response in life-threatening crises. If the hyper-aroused energy state of the fight/flight/freeze reaction is not resolved and discharged, its pattern remains trapped like a vortex in the nervous system and the victim endlessly relives the experience and its attendant emotions. Animals instinctively release this energy physiologically, that is at the body level, for example through shivering. We humans, with our rational inhibitions, are less attuned to our instincts and so more prone to becoming ensnared by this vicious circle (Levine 1997).

Having cancer unfortunately gives rise to multiple occasions for traumatic experiences. Indeed, Goldie and Desmarais (2005, p.11) talk of the 'shell-shock of cancer'. The diagnosis may be given in an abrupt and unfeeling way; there may be frightening memories of other family members dying in great pain from cancer; the ill person has to face her own mortality; surgery may be mutilating; radiotherapy and especially chemotherapy may cause severe side-effects and complications such as septicaemia; clinical progression may bring terrifying complications such as haemorrhages or severe breathlessness; and memories of past traumatic events may be re-activated. PTSD is more likely to be diagnosed in survivors who live long enough for the condition to be recognised. However, I wonder if some cases of extreme distress in those very close to dying may not be a reactivation of past traumas from childhood that the patient has kept hidden; as he approaches death, his psychological defences break down and the long-suppressed memories surface with their attendant anguish. So-called 'terminal restlessness', which is more a clinical observation than a diagnosis, may relate to this on occasion. By this stage the patient is usually beyond talking and high doses of injected tranquillisers may be urgently needed to relieve the extreme distress of his final hours.

One group where PTSD may get missed is war veterans. Many patients referred for palliative care will have lived through the Second World War and may have had horrifying experiences (developing what used to be called battle fatigue). Over the years they may have come to accept their continuing nightmares and flashbacks as an inevitable part of their lives, such that they don't even mention it. It is, therefore, well worth enquiring since treatment is possible.

What helps those not so close to death? People with PTSD get trapped in reliving their trauma repeatedly and so re-traumatising themselves. Hence inviting them to go into their experience and relive it repeatedly can be counterproductive and cause unnecessary distress. One useful technique, whether for PTSD or for recent acute traumatic experiences, is to teach them a 'safe place' visualisation. This is similar to the first visualisation described in Chapter 5, with the following differences:

- The patient is asked to recall a place where she felt safe and at peace. Often this turns out to be in nature – on a beach or in a secluded valley, for example – but it can be anywhere that brings a sense of security.

- She is asked to bring to mind the place using each of the senses, so making the recollection as vivid as possible, and to spend time quietly experiencing the peacefulness of this sanctuary.

- Before leaving her safe place, she is asked to focus on an 'anchor', something she can touch in the visualisation such as the bark of a tree or the feel of sand, or perhaps a word. Whenever she returns to this sanctuary, bringing to mind the anchor will help her enter the experience again, especially if she is in a distressed state.

This can be used whenever the patient experiences trauma feelings, or, which is yet more useful, as a regular meditation to reduce background anxiety and as a prophylactic. In a similar way, the muscle relaxation exercises described in Chapter 5 may be helpful as may meditations where the patient simply focuses on awareness of his breathing (LeShan 1999). Support by palliative care clinicians needs to be just that – supportive; it is about trying to create the ambience of a 'safe place' in the hospice or at home. This is to do with containing anxiety rather than asking patients to go into their fear with resultant re-traumatisation. Where practicable, a problem-solving approach may be useful, particularly by assisting patients in switching their focus away from their helplessness feelings towards re-empowerment. They may have more manageable anxieties about going home, making a will or seeing a long-lost relative, all of which can be addressed with the assistance of the palliative care staff caring for them.

There are several therapeutic approaches to PTSD such as CBT, and somatic experiencing (SE), which focuses on body sensations as the traumatic event is recalled (Levine 1997). One well-researched, effective and widely used method is eye movement desensitisation and reprocessing (EMDR) (Shapiro and Forrest 2004). An American psychologist, Francine Shapiro, discovered that rapid lateral eye movements or other lateralising stimuli, such as alternate hand tapping or sounds in each ear sequentially, can help to alleviate PTSD symptoms. EMDR seems to release the frozen memories and emotions from their trapped state and allows their processing and integration to be completed. It has been likened to rapid eye movement (REM) sleep which facilitates a similar progression. EMDR should only be carried out by trained practitioners as part of a comprehensive treatment programme that includes psychotherapy. It may work rapidly; sometimes only a few sessions are needed. Social workers on palliative care units may know of trained practitioners; if not, organisations such as the British Association for Counselling and Psychotherapy (BACP) will have lists of EMDR therapists.

THE HUMAN FAMILY

When I was on holiday in Trinidad, I drove out along a peninsula of land to where a Hindu temple had been built out onto the sea. On the shore was an open-air crematorium. I saw a body burning on a pyre of wood with relatives standing nearby; a little way off was another pyre, by then an oblong heap of ashes. I had never seen this before and the exposed nature of this ritual came as something of a shock. Cremation in England is such a discreet, hidden affair. I found myself rather admiring the openness of the Hindu approach. I was encountering one aspect of the diversity of customs worldwide in relation to dying.

The terms used to describe human diversity are not exact, overlap and reflect the complexity of this subject (d'Ardenne and Mahtani 1989). 'Race' is usually taken to refer to physical characteristics, particularly of skin colour, even though such traits do not actually define a group. For instance, among those who identify themselves as 'black' there may be individuals who are lighter-skinned than some who call themselves 'white' (Reber and Reber 2001). It is important never to make assumptions about how individuals will define themselves racially. There are, therefore, cultural traits that attend racial identity. What, then, does culture mean? It relates to a group, be this a nation, religion, race or custom and it describes their shared beliefs, artistic heritage, practices and so on. Ethnicity refers to any group, often a minority, with a common cultural tradition and identity.

It is also true that every person we meet is different from us in some way. Prejudice, therefore, may manifest, for example, as racism, ageism, sexism, homophobia and anti-semitism. On occasion, I have met people with cancer phobia – they fear they might catch cancer like an infection and so shun those with this illness as if they were lepers. Clinicians are not immune from such fears. Goldie and Desmarais (2005, p.27) describe a cancer hospital where the staff 'would not drink out of clean cups previously used by the patients'. People whose cancer has resulted from their life-style may be stigmatised. Patients with AIDS, which may present with disfiguring skin malignancies such as Kaposi's sarcoma, have particularly been the target of this prejudice.

Hospices will vary widely in the ethnic diversity of the patients they care for; those in districts of large cities with high immigrant populations such as London or Birmingham will obviously receive more minority ethnic patients. However, they may still be under-represented compared with the local white population, perhaps because they are younger on average and so less prone to developing cancer. Palliative care provision is not so much to the fore in some cultures, so that many from these backgrounds may approach illness and dying in their traditional ways, perhaps not aware that a palliative care resource is available. Language may be a barrier, too, in communicating their needs to their general practitioner.

Counselling skills use in communicating with those of different ethnicities must, of course, be adapted to each individual. For many, counselling isn't part of their culture. So, getting some background information about their culture before seeing patients is obviously useful; but, at the same time, hardly anyone conforms exactly to their cultural norms. Therefore it is important to find out from individuals what their requirements are with respect to their beliefs and practices. They will probably welcome your interest. We have constantly to question our assumptions. For example, many Muslim women do not shake hands with men. This can lead to a topsy-turvey situation. When I meet Muslim women, I do not shake hands with them. They, however, as a mark of courtesy to English culture, and perhaps because so many white men in England have shaken their hand, do actually put out their hand to shake mine.

Body language varies, too. Thus, southern Europeans stand closer to others when conversing than their northern counterparts. The thumbs up sign means all's well in the USA but in some Islamic countries it has sexual connotations. Be aware of eye contact. In Arab and Latin American populations, this is generally greater than in Europe, but in other cultures such as India and Japan, it is less – a stare might be seen as a showing aggression or superiority. The person you are talking to will give you cues as to the level of eye contact she feels comfortable with.

Remember also that other cultures do not necessarily share the Western view that the individual is pre-eminent. India has a more collectivist cultural view, for example. We in the West may think patients are entitled to information about their illness no matter what their family may say to the contrary. Indian patients may not find this so easy to deal with and may not leap at the opportunity.

For patients who can't speak English, it's not usually a good idea to use family members to translate conversations requiring a counselling approach. They may not understand you fully themselves and they may, unknown to you, censor your comments and questions either to prevent distress to the patient or because it is not culturally appropriate to broach certain topics such as prognosis. It may be, too, that the only family member available is a 14-year-old; it would not be appropriate to expect a teenager to carry the burden of such serious discussions. It is better to use advocates. These are employed by NHS Trusts not only to be translators but also to be advocates for patients and their individual cultural needs. Apart from accurate translation, they can also advise on the cultural suitability of questions around breaking bad news. When working with a patient and advocate, it is important to look at the patient when speaking and when the advocate is replying on his behalf. This helps to maintain contact despite the language barrier.

Different cultures will interpret illness very differently. Thus what is conceptualised as depression in the West is interpreted more in terms of physical symptoms on the Indian sub-continent. Schizophrenia is far more commonly diagnosed in Afro-Caribbeans living in Great Britain than in those living in the Caribbean.

Attitudes to life-threatening illness vary widely. There has been a radical shift of viewpoint in the West in recent decades with a move to open discussion of the diagnosis and prognosis. This is not so in many other cultures and it is important to be sensitive to this. For Hindus, and for the Chinese, to talk about dying is considered bad luck with the possibility that it might hasten the patient's death. I was told of one dramatic incident concerning a Chinese man, unable to speak English, who was admitted to a hospice dying of cancer. When his wife found out about his condition, she went and pulled all the buttons off his jacket, signifying to him that he was dead, and then left him. He did indeed die shortly afterwards and his carers were hampered by not being able to talk with him about his feelings concerning what had happened.

In Judaism, all life is considered precious. Some Jews interpret this strictly and consider it essential to fight for life no matter what, even if the patient is terminally ill. Many take a more relaxed view. One woman I looked after was close to dying from cancer and unable to speak. Her brother was insistent on her being transferred to an acute hospital for further treatment and wanted to contact a consultant there immediately to take over her care. I was in a dilemma. I could see she was going to die soon, and I felt any move would cause her physical distress and might actually hasten her death, but how could I also respect the cultural imperatives here, especially as the patient couldn't tell us herself what she wanted? I spent over an hour discussing this with her brother. He felt passionately about this issue. Much of the time I was listening to him explaining his view and perhaps this was helpful to him – he had been heard. I focused on the inevitability of her death no matter what treatment she received and pointed out that I would have referred her to hospital myself if I thought there was any chance of this helping. We agreed to call in a rabbi. He felt that every reasonable effort had been made in the treatment of the patient and that it was not necessary to refer her to hospital. The woman's brother accepted this and the patient died soon afterwards.

Differences in ethnicity may affect transference and countertransference reactions between patient and clinician – beliefs, prejudices, values and feelings about race may all come into play. Thus, I am white, fair-haired and have a middle-class English accent. I may be talking to an Afro-Caribbean man with a Jamaican accent and a name that was given to his forebears by a white slave-master. I belong to a nation that enslaved this man's ancestors. While I am not personally to blame, I may feel a sense of guilt about this shameful episode and so feel an inner pressure to make amends by trying harder to help him. He, in turn, may find he likes me but at the same time he may be aware of feelings about the oppression of his people by my ancestors and so he is cautious in what he says to me; he may also have had bad experiences with other doctors. Our histories – of slavery and imperialism – collide in the field between us. Awareness helps us move beyond the past without forgetting it.

CHAPTER 10

Spiritual Distress

SOUL, SPIRIT AND PSYCHE

These words are used in many ways, sometimes as synonyms, sometimes distinctively. 'Soul' comes from the Old English *sawol*, which may, in turn, come from a Germanic root meaning 'sea'. 'Spirit' comes from Latin *spiritus*, meaning 'breath'. Thus the elements of water and air have been invoked, both essential to life. Some of the ways soul and spirit have been conceptualised are as follows:

- the essence of a person
- the life force
- an immortal ethereal entity
- consciousness.

To complicate matters further, the Greek word *psyche* was used to describe soul, mind and self, and also meant a butterfly. Nowadays, the word soul is coming back into psychology (Hillman 1992). Integrative psychosynthesis (Robertson 1997) uses spirit to refer to the transcendent, to spiritual experiences. It sees soul as the meeting place between spirit and the body – where the spirit becomes incarnate and the body becomes sacred. Its associations include depth, richness, imagination, feeling and beauty. Thus, we may speak of soul music or a soulful piece of writing. Soul may inhabit tragedy as well, something familiar to anyone working with the dying. A useful analogy is of a tree (the soul) with its branches in the air (spirit) and its roots in the earth (the body).

RECOGNITION

Spiritual distress is about estrangement from the essence of our being. It is not surprising that the prospect of death will highlight this. Spiritual distress is under-recognised in the dying and may be confused with psychological distress (Heyse-Moore 1996). In this context, 'spiritual' is not the same as 'religious'. Spirituality is about a person's relationship with the core of who she is and, as such, is a term that can be used by everyone, whatever their belief. Religion is an expression of spirituality according to a pre-existing set of beliefs, such as Christianity or Islam.

Recognising spiritual distress requires looking at symptoms with bifocal vision; first the literal, physical presentation and, second, the symbolic level. We talk about a person dying of a broken heart, for example, where the *double entendre* is obvious. But what about breathlessness and dying of a lack of the breath of life? To have a stroke implies being struck – a divine blow. Pain is a physical warning signal, but at another level religious traditions have much to say about it: Christians talk of uniting their suffering with that of Christ; one of the Buddha's four noble truths states that the root of suffering is attachment; Muslims invoke *mektoub*, the will of Allah.

A Zulu proverb says: a person is a person because of people. We need each other, we need to relate to each other, and in depth. If this goes, if he treats the other as an 'it', perhaps because he has been hurt in the past, the soul goes out of his contacts with other people. He may say he feels isolated, lonely, depressed. Again, the symptom points to the loss of soul.

And then there are specific symptoms of soul pain:

* *Meaninglessness*: this is exemplified by Macbeth's lament, to which I have already alluded briefly, on hearing of the death of his queen (Shakespeare 1905, pp.867–8):

    Tomorrow and tomorrow and tomorrow,
    Creeps in this petty pace from day to day,
    To the last syllable of recorded time:
    And all our yesterdays have lighted fools
    The way to dusty death. Out, out, brief candle!
    Life's but a walking shadow, a poor player
    That struts and frets his hour upon the stage,
    And then is heard no more; it is a tale
    Told by an idiot, full of sound and fury,
    Signifying nothing.

- *Anguish*: the experience of Jesus in the garden of Gethsemane, in Luke 22:41–4, when in terror and anguish he sweated blood as he faced the prospect of his imminent, violent death (Jones 1966, p.118) speaks to this. Some people close to dying seem to experience a similar soul distress even when they have no physical symptoms.

- *Duality*: the dying person feels cut off from herself, her loved ones and the world around her. This is alluded to in Philip Pullman's novel *Northern Lights* (1995) where every character has a daemon, an attendant spirit, in the form of an animal – a kind of soul figure. A person and his daemon are, literally, inseparable. For them to try to part causes intolerable pain. The evil General Oblation Board cuts children apart from their daemon, so-called intercision. The children that survive become lost, half-children, split off from their life spirit.

- *Inner darkness*: this was famously described by St John of the Cross (1976) as the dark night of the soul. His phrase aptly captures the feeling of blindness, of walking in the dark, of losing ones bearings and of aloneness that dying people may experience.

Religious distress occurs when a person comes into conflict with his previously faithfully held religious beliefs, or when he has internalised an excessively judgemental or moralistic view of his religion – Catholic guilt is a well-known example.

What helps then? We need to remember that although many patients do not have a formal religious belief and may not wish to see a minister, nevertheless, they may be experiencing a crisis of meaning as described above. So, it may fall to any clinician to address these issues, no matter what her personal beliefs are.

First, the quality of your presence plays an important part. Here is an unusual and vivid example about an old woman from south India (Harvey and Matousek 1994, pp. 267–8):

> She had suffered tremendously when young, lost many members of her family in a tragic accident and finally come to a state of suicidal depression. She went to Ramana Maharshi, who happened to be alone in the small room where he gave darshan, and started to cry, telling him the story of her life. The Maharshi said nothing and went on saying nothing. Slowly the woman stopped crying, stopped talking and just sat with him, gazing into his eyes. She told me that at that moment,

light filled the room, and her heart opened as if by the most delicate spear, running right through the centre. This meeting opened in her a bliss she never dreamt could exist, streaming from his compassion.

This presence may be silent: a relative or member of staff sitting quietly with a dying person, perhaps holding his hand. We return again to Cicely Saunders' phrase: watch with me.

It can be seen that much of what has already been described as psychological process and the use of counselling skills, also addresses issues of soul pain. Indeed guided imagery as used in psychosynthesis is intended to access the transpersonal dimension. The visualisations of a country scene described in Chapter 5 are a case in point. Though it is apparently a natural landscape, each element can also be seen as a metaphor. Thus, trees are a symbol of life, the wind reminds us of the spirit, the sun speaks of illumination and the lake of stillness. If a person is imagined walking by the lake, this may represent a source of wisdom for the imagineer. When I did this visualisation with one woman, I remember being struck by how the anxious distress on her face gradually dissolved into calmness, and the empty, hungry look gave way to plenitude. For a little, her consciousness was transformed. Afterwards, her whole approach to her fatal illness changed; she became more accepting and trusting and spent time preparing herself and her family for her forthcoming death.

It's worth taking note of any spiritual symbols the patient has in her room – images of Christ, the Buddha or Krishna, for example, or perhaps the prayer beads used in Christianity, Islam or Buddhism. One of the most frequent, often unremarked, is the St Christopher medallion worn round the neck, invoking the saint who carried weary pilgrims safely across deep waters. Usually, these bring comfort. One woman with advanced cancer, however, had multiple chains around her neck with images of Christ, the Virgin Mary, St Christopher and Padre Pio among others. Pinned to her nightgown was a forest of prayer cards, blessed medallions and further religious images. It didn't take much insight on my part to tell that she was very frightened and was invoking these figures to protect her from her terrors of death.

If a minister or chaplain sees a patient, potentially he has a dual role. On the one hand, he may approach the patient in the ways described above, especially if he is seeing someone with no spiritual practice or belief. This was summed up by a patient who told me that the chaplain had visited – he had found it a good experience and was especially pleased that God had not been mentioned once. Nevertheless, the big questions may appear: Why me? Is there a God? How can there be a God with so much suffering? Is there any meaning to life? Is there an after-life? Who am I? Why am I here? Who am I becoming? Suddenly, these queries become all too relevant with death nearing. They are not, however, just matters for debate at the rational level, important though that is. They carry feelings too, often strong feelings, which need a voice and which may take a different view to a dry piece of logic.

On the other hand, the patient may want to avail herself of the rituals of a specifically religious ministry. Buddhist chants, lighting the Jewish seven-branched candlestick, the Muslim call to prayer, the Christian sacraments: all of these may be deeply comforting to their respective followers.

Rituals can also be created according to individual need and this is something that can be discussed with the patient if he so wishes. Some form of forgiveness is a frequent theme and deep need. This may be an acknowledgement of a past wrong, or the wish to be reconciled with another who has wronged the patient. It can happen, however, that patients experience such intense shame that this is indicative of the destructive messages which they took in as part of a traumatic childhood rather than any actual misdemeanour. In this case, there is a journey towards discovering that they were *not* wrong, rather it is *they* who were harmed. Here, the chaplain needs the skills to distinguish where rituals of absolution and where counselling skills are appropriate, or indeed if both are needed.

Rituals are, in fact, happening all the time in hospices, even if they are not necessarily noted as such. A partner brings in flowers or fruit; a grand-daughter brings in a picture she has drawn for her grandpa; there is a bottle of champagne on the bedside table to celebrate an anniversary or a cake to mark a birthday; a couple listen to a favourite piece of music together. I have a picture of a man with advanced cancer sitting with his daughter, who is in her wedding dress, and his new son-in-law – the difference is that the reception took place in his palliative care unit because he was too frail to travel to the church. Some couples decide to renew their wedding vows. One couple decided to get married in the palliative care unit where she was an in-patient. I remember being moved by the care taken by the nurses in helping her to prepare – her dress, her hair, the flowers. There may be reunions with family members not seen for decades. Families may even independently bring in faith healers, who carry out their own ritual laying on of hands.

Furthermore, the actions of clinical staff have a ritual element: nurses washing patients, changing their dressings, feeding them, turning them in bed or laying them out when they have died; doctors examining patients and treating them. All of these can be done mechanically and soullessly, or the opposite, personally and soulfully. I remember watching a nurse help a patient out of bed, such a simple task. I was struck by the care she took in turning back the bedclothes, in helping the woman to move to the edge of the bed, swing her legs over and so on, one gentle step at a time, until this frail old lady was standing – it all seemed so effortless – while the nurse solicitously smoothed down her nightdress so that she looked her best when she walked to her chair. The nurse's message to this woman was, to my mind, you are still you however ill you are. One might call this a form of body therapy – and then recall that body, mind and spirit are intimately interconnected.

And what about prayer? Its literal meaning is to ask earnestly or to beg. Most people pray in times of desperation, whatever their usual beliefs. Indeed, I imagine that if silent prayers could be made visible like smoke, then dense, mutely imploring clouds would be seen rising from hospices. Many who pray will anxiously beg for a cure or even a remission. Perhaps the greatest gift they, or indeed any of us, can receive is to be able to accept their condition with its uncertain future. Various studies have been carried out on the effects of prayer on illnesses with variable results. Perhaps, though, these miss the point. Prayer is not an ethereal pharmacotherapy dispensed under controlled conditions. It is about the individual's relationship with the depths of her being. Whether she sees this in terms of Christ, Yahweh, Brahma or Allah, she is praying to her creator, the source of her being, who keeps her in existence from moment to moment. She is safe, even in the psalmist's valley of the shadow of death. No wonder people pray.

Meditation, by contrast, does not necessarily carry religious or spiritual connotations and so can be useful to anyone no matter what their belief. It is particularly valuable as part of a counselling approach in helping patients who are anxious or restless to find calmness. The examples given in Chapter 5 are forms of meditation and there are numerous books detailing other methods (LeShan 1999). From a spiritual perspective, the meditative principle of self-awareness or mindfulness runs through many religious traditions – Christianity, Hinduism, Sufism and Buddhism, for example. What they highlight is that the experience of stillness, though not easily come by, speaks to the core of our being. Practitioners talk of the ineffable, of fullness, timelessness, lightness, space, silence, ease and clarity in trying to describe something they find to be beyond mere words. For them, meditation and prayer are two sides of the same coin. This is a personal, private area and they may choose not to speak about their rich, inner life even when dying.

I have talked to patients who have had near-death experiences (NDEs). They have reported the life-changing effect this had on them: the abolition of their fear of death, their meeting with a loving presence and their certainty of an after-life. One person, however, told me of a more ambiguous, frightening experience and this fear was re-evoked as she approached death. Clearly it was important to know this to provide her with appropriate psychological and pastoral support. However, those close to death may not tell us what they are experiencing. I believe there may be much happening, even in those who appear unconscious. They do respond to what is occurring around them but they do so subtly through changes in breathing or heart rate, a slight movement of a hand, flushing, inarticulate sounds and so on. Mindell (1994, pp.8–10), a psychotherapist, describes a remarkable story of being asked to see an old man in hospital who had been semi-comatose for months and continually groaned and yelled incoherently. Mindell entrained himself with the man by groaning in synchrony and by squeezing his hand in time with his breathing and heartbeat. After 20 minutes, the man began to speak – his words were slurred but comprehensible. He could see a big ship, he said, but there was no way he was getting on it as it was going on vacation and he had to go to work. Prompted by Mindell, he looked and saw that angels were driving the ship and that it was a free ride; they were beckoning him to join them. Mindell suggested to him that he think it over – what about a vacation? He could always come back. Mindell went off to see another client and returned half an hour later. The man had died. He had decided to take that vacation.

What are we to make of this account? To the atheist, this is nothing but the hallucinations, the psychic debris, of a dying man. To the psychotherapist, these are archetypal emanations of the unconscious. Angels are, metaphorically, messengers, here portending the patient's imminent death, and the ship is a powerful symbol of transition, from life to death. To those with a spiritual belief, this is a vision of divine envoys sent to accompany the dying man on his journey to Paradise. Each reader will have his own view. Where, perhaps, there can be a meeting point is through stepping outside the interpretations and tasting the flavour of the story itself – powerful, affecting and strange. Next time you are with a dying person, whether she is semi- or unconscious, stop and consider that dramas such as the above story may be playing out within her unknown to the outside world.

CHAPTER 11

The Sick Psyche

This chapter is about the use of counselling skills in certain psychopathologies likely to be encountered in palliative care. While the term 'psychopathology' implies a disease process in a similar manner to physical illnesses, it is worth remembering that the root meaning of *psyche-pathos-logos* is 'the speech of the suffering soul', a point elaborated by Hillman (1992) who views these maladies as expressions in their own right of the archetypal depths of the psyche rather than simply as neuronal malfunctions.

GENERAL STRATEGIES

- Use an empathic supportive approach. People with fragmented psyches struggle to cope with being confronted.

- Be attentive to boundaries. Alcoholics, drug abusers or those with a borderline personality disorder, for example, have difficulty maintaining their own boundaries. They may act out their distress through self-harm, getting drunk or aggressive behaviour. It is important, therefore, to agree boundaries with them and to be consistent in maintaining them.

- Splitting as part of a fractured personality may be reflected in the potential for splitting among staff. The patient may insist on being looked after by one nurse who is considered brilliant, while the others are rejected as incompetent. It is vital, therefore, for staff to communicate well and to have a clear, agreed strategy for dealing with such behaviour; in other words to model a united approach to the patient rather than collude with his dividedness.

- Enlist the aid of professionals trained in working with these people. Often this will involve psychiatric input since these patients are frequently on long-term psychotropic medication and may have become disturbed because they have not been taking their drugs.

SPECIFICS
Alcoholism

This is not uncommon among patients admitted to hospices. As a rule, it is better not to suggest that they dry out. This would cause considerable distress and would achieve little or nothing in someone who has not long to live anyway. Most alcoholics will simply continue their present level of intake. Care must obviously be taken with other sedative drugs. One elderly woman in-patient drank about three-quarters of a bottle of gin a day. She was able to converse lucidly despite taking morphine as well and made it clear she did not want to talk about her feelings. During times of stress, such as deaths in her bay, her gin consumption increased, sometimes doubling. This was her chosen way of dealing with her emotions and she continued in this fashion until she died.

Borderline personality disorder

Over the years, in the various hospices I have worked in, there have been a number of memorable patients or family members who have been labelled as 'difficult' by staff. With hindsight it is clear that, some, at least, of these exhibited behaviour that was consistent with a borderline personality disorder (BPD), but were not recognised as such at the time. Identification is important, not only so that the individual can receive appropriate care, but also for staff, since people with BPD can evoke strong counter-transference reactions with the risk of splitting in the hospice team.

Some features of BPD include the following (American Psychiatric Association 2000, p.301):

- relationships

    o instability (alternating between idealisation and condemnation)

    o intense fears of abandonment

- mood
  - affective instability
  - feelings of emptiness
  - outbursts of anger
  - paranoid thoughts
  - dissociation
- behaviour
  - impulsivity (eating disorders, drug abuse, overspending)
  - suicidal or self-harming behaviour
- identity instability.

Clinicians working with BPD patients or relatives may experience unexpectedly intense countertransference feelings in a number of ways, such as anger ('She is so frustrating to work with!'), sadness ('What a heartbreaking story'), helplessness ('I don't know how to help her'), euphoria ('She is so appreciative of the help I'm giving her') or fear ('I'm scared of her violent temper'). Projective identification may be part of this. As different members of staff work with this individual, these feelings may diffuse into the whole team. There may be acrimonious arguments at ward meetings as to how to deal with this awkward person. The team is beginning to reflect the patient's fragmented psyche; hence the need for a united approach that maintains the limits the patient has difficulty keeping. Clinicians trained in psychological therapies and familiar with BPD, such as social workers, will have a central role to play in guiding the rest of the team in this task. As an example, one relative with features of BPD used to drink heavily and leave empty whisky bottles around the unit; or he would arrive drunk and was, at times, verbally aggressive. It was necessary to meet with him. We discussed his behaviour with him and he had an opportunity to ventilate his understandable distress at the prospect of his partner dying. We continued to meet with him frequently to support him. He realised the effects of his behaviour, and we were able to agree boundaries with him – visits to the unit required that he was not aggressively drunk, and that he would not leave his empties around. He acquiesced, and from time to time tested the boundaries as people with BPD do. But we continued to meet with him and reiterate our team commitment to the limits we had agreed and he was able to cooperate to a workable degree.

Treatment of BPD requires specialist input – approaches include long-term psychotherapy, forms of CBT such a dialectical behaviour therapy and medication (antidepressants or antipsychotics). People with BPD often suffer from PTSD following childhood abuse and hence may benefit from EMDR. Obviously these long-term therapies are not feasible in dying patients. In practice, the usual input is a combination of empathic support and medication to stabilise mood.

Psychoses

Psychotic patients lose the ability to distinguish between inner and outer realities, so that the two become mingled. This may be in the form of delusions (demonstrably false beliefs) or hallucinations (most often visual or auditory). For example, one man I talked to with advanced cancer was acutely paranoid. He thought the nurses were dressed in traditional Dutch costumes and the doctors in prison guard uniforms. He was certain they were out to kill him. It was not surprising he refused all care.

Challenging such beliefs directly will only make matters worse – the patient will think you are in league with the others who are out to harm him. Instead, concentrate on getting alongside him, trying to enter his world and see it from his perspective. After all, if you think there is a conspiracy to kill you, it would be perfectly consistent to be suspicious of anyone who comes to talk to you. But, as a clinician, you can say to the patient: 'That must be very alarming' or 'I imagine that must have been very frightening for you'. It is often possible in this way to maintain empathic contact with the patient, though it may be very slow, delicate work – almost anything you say can be misperceived as an attack. 'How are you?' might bring the riposte: 'Why do you want to know?' for example. There may be a particular staff member or relative the patient trusts, will talk to and from whom he will accept medication. Some patients may be quietly delusional in a way that does not distress them, but, for the majority, their psychotic symptoms are accompanied by much emotional distress, often paranoid in tone. For these latter, antipsychotic medication is usually needed; as these drugs begin to take effect, over the ensuing days it becomes more possible to work with them psychologically and they are often able to look back on their delusions and recognise them as such.

I was taught a lesson in the importance of a slow, empathic approach when I was asked to see a patient who had a manic psychosis secondary to her cancer. My attempts to stem her rapid and unending stream of ever-changing thoughts flowing through her mindscape and to persuade her to focus her reflections were met with increasing aggression, culminating in an assault. Never again!

Compulsory detention?

A patient may in principle, if seriously disturbed mentally, be admitted to a psychiatric unit compulsorily if her own health or safety is at risk or for the protection of others. This is under Section 2 of the Mental Health Act 1983 (Puri *et al.* 1996, p.399). In practice I have never had to do this and, from conversations with colleagues, it is a rare occurrence in palliative care units. Almost always it is possible to talk the patient down and to persuade her to accept anti-psychotic medication. Rarely, in a crisis, if a psychotic individual is extremely agitated and a danger to herself or others, it may be necessary to administer a tranquilliser without her consent – she is, in fact, not able to give it at this point. While this is recognised as acceptable clinical practice in an emergency, it is still important, when she is calmer, to find out if she wishes to talk through her feelings about what happened to her.

Delirium

This is characterised by clouding of consciousness, confusion, disorientation, varying agitation and sleepiness, memory loss and often hallucinations, delusions and illusions (for example, mistaking shadows for people). It can be caused by a wide variety of physical conditions such as brain metastases, strokes, drug and alcohol withdrawal, drug toxicity, kidney failure, raised blood calcium levels and pneumonia. It is common in palliative care. By the very nature of the condition, the usual counselling skills will not be helpful, but a more body-centred approach may be of use:

- Medically, correct any correctable cause of delirium.
- A quiet single room is better than a bed in a bay.
- Subdued lighting but enough to avoid shadows.

- Family, volunteers or staff to sit with the patient and, if so wished, hold his hand.

- Familiar objects from home around the patient, including a newspaper with today's date.

- A clock with a clearly visible face and showing the right time. So often, I have found the patients' own watch has stopped and is showing the wrong date.

- Television may be better avoided as the source of further delusional ideas.

- It can be difficult to understand what a delirious patient is saying because of his slurred speech and confusion of ideas, but it is important to try since he may, in the midst of his bewildered, fogged state, be trying very hard to communicate with you.

- It may be all you can do is to repeat the incoherent words or phrases the patient is saying as a way of indicating you are listening. Some hospice staff have a particular gift for being able to understand the slurred speech being offered. This feedback may sometimes help patients clarify what they want to say. If she groans inarticulately, you can make a soft sound in sympathy.

- Try entraining with the patient – for example, breathing in synchrony with him, blinking when he does, moving slightly in correspondence with his movements. This may increase your empathic resonance.

- You can also comment on what is happening with the patient's body: 'I notice that you're moving your arm'; 'You made a face just then'; 'You just took a deep breath'.

- If any clinical procedures are being carried out, talk to the patient and tell him what you are doing.

Dementia

For people with dementia, too, familiarity is important in helping them keep in contact with their environment. Conversations may, on the surface, have some semblance of normality – demented people have normal levels of consciousness. It is their forgetfulness, when they repeat the same question five minutes later, that renders counselling input difficult and frustrating. Furthermore, there may be deterioration in emotional control, use of language and understanding of what is being said. Since dementia is a gradual process, the clinician has to keep modifying her responses to the patient to keep pace with changes in the level of his understanding. This is the case with breaking bad news. Early on in the dementing process the patient may still be able to comprehend and retain information about his illness. Later on, he may not. As previously discussed, it would be cruel to break bad news repeatedly every time he forgets and asks again – he would suffer the ensuing emotional distress over and over again. How, then, can an assessment be made of what to say? The Mental Capacity Act 2005 (Mukherjee and Foster 2008) gives useful parameters. An individual lacks the capacity to give consent – in this case to discussing his diagnosis – if he cannot:

- understand the information
- retain this knowledge
- make use of the information or assess its pros and cons
- communicate this to another person.

This is decision-specific, that is it relates a particular occasion. This is important in early stages of dementia where mental capacity will vary from day to day.

So how can we respond to queries about their health from those with dementia who lack mental capacity? In the first place it will most likely be difficult for them to formulate a detailed question. Rather, their query may be: 'What's happening to me?' or 'How am I getting on?' In response, we need to acknowledge and empathise with their concerns. We need particularly to find ways of communicating warmth and support through our presence to them, whatever their individual anxieties – pain, where their partner is, why they have a catheter, when can they go home and so on. Knowing that they will forget your answers, it is more the tone of your voice, calmness, unhurriedness, attention and patience which will help. It may feel strange to avoid openness and even to divert their attention sometimes, the very opposite of what I have so far been advocating. This is, however, in the spirit of the ethical principle of non-maleficence, to do no harm.

While forgetfulness may shield a patient from the distress of knowing she is dying, the same does not apply for her family. They have to watch the gradual destruction of their loved one's personality as well as bear the knowledge of her forthcoming death, a double blow, especially as personal contact is so important at this time. They may perceive her as not being there any more, as having died while the shell of her body remains alive. Bereavement counselling support and the chance to process their feelings about this will be particularly relevant. An analogy some relatives with a spiritual belief may find helpful is that of a driver in a car. The car is not working properly – the steering is broken, the windscreen cracked. However, the person inside, her essence, remains the same even though she cannot communicate properly with the outside world.

CHAPTER 12

Staff Support

I remember a doctor who was part of the doctors' mess when I was a junior house officer. She seemed to have a talkative, extrovert personality, but I recalled how she was when attending a patient in cardiac arrest – shaking visibly, agitated, tense and anxious. A couple of days later I learned she had committed suicide. I never knew her story. While it is likely that she had previous personal issues, it is clear that the stresses inherent in working with sick people were significant for her as they are for any clinical discipline. Interestingly, no lessons were learned from her death. No-one at a managerial level considered it might be important to assess how her colleagues were coping with their workloads or their feelings about her death. Her memory disappeared into corporate denial.

What about care of the dying? A specialist registrar in palliative medicine wrote about her experience of depression (*BMA News* 2007). She described her distorted sense of reality, inability to make decisions, breathlessness, shaking, pains, suicidal images and loss of memory. It was a terrifying experience, but the outcome was different. She got help. Her therapies included time off work, counselling, antidepressants, and ensuring she looked after herself, especially through support from friends, and exercise. This story summarises the various aspects of staff support which will be considered in this chapter.

Working with dying people can be stressful. This would seem obvious and yet I have heard it denied by some working in palliative care who say it is no different to any other clinical specialty. Nevertheless, each area of health care carries its own particular stresses – the busy accident and emergency department, crises on the labour ward, or intensive care units where lives hang by a thread. It's true that palliative care does not have

these factors to contend with, but there are others. All the patients die –
this doesn't happen in any other clinical specialty and it runs counter to the
received wisdom of health care training which is predicated on cure.
Patients and their families may be in extreme emotional distress. They may
suffer severe resistant pain and other symptoms. They may be in despair
and suicidal. They may have appalling, foul-smelling, ulcerating cancers.
They may haemorrhage to death. These and many other stressors, while
they may occur in other branches of clinical care, are compounded by the
difference of approach in palliative care whereby life-saving measures
(which can function as a way of denying the reality of an impending death)
are not automatically invoked and where clinicians spend time listening to
the distress of the dying and entering into their world. Yes, there are
stresses in this work even if they tend to be of the slow-burn variety as
opposed to the rush of acute specialties (Vachon 1995).

Of the different clinical disciplines, doctors are especially vulnerable in
this respect (Feld and Heyse-Moore 2006) with high rates of burnout,
depression, suicide and alcoholism, and little formal support. In striking
contrast, social workers who are counselling patients have to have regular
supervision from a trained supervisor.

What, then, motivates clinicians to work in such a demanding area?
While this will vary with individuals and their discipline, some initial
answers might include:

- I'm interested in symptom control.
- It's an area where I can be a proper nurse.
- I enjoy the opportunity to use my counselling skills.
- I want to carry out research into pain management.
- I like working in a small unit where you get to know
  everybody and there's enough staff.
- As a minister I feel I have a vocation to the dying.

Underlying this, however, and often unexpressed at job interviews for fear
of being thought soft, is, surely, a compassion for the suffering of the dying
and a wish to alleviate this. Perhaps an individual had a family member
who died of cancer in distressing circumstances and this motivated him to
want to work with the dying. At a deeper level, he may have experienced
significant illness, whether physical or psychological, in his life and he

wishes to bring to others the care and support that was brought to him –
this is the archetype of the Wounded Healer who draws on his own sufferings to understand better the sufferings of others.

There may be more unconscious motivations too. There is, for
example, the compulsive carer who gives to others the love that she never
received. And, death is frightening. One way for clinicians to control their
fear is to control the pain, the psychological distress, the family suffering,
the loss of body functions and so on through nursing and medical
procedures. Death is seemingly made safe and sanitised. Furthermore,
every time a clinician and patient meet, there is the potential for a polarity
to be set up. Psychologically, the clinician assumes the role of healer, the
patient that of the dying one. There is a split which keeps the clinician
'safe' because the patient is embodying the dying role so the clinician
doesn't have to address that potential within himself.

Motivations, then, may be more complicated than would at first
appear. As well as this, clinicians are just as prone as anyone else to
developing psychological ailments or to having had a past history of these
conditions. Anxiety, depression, stress-related illness, family conflict,
bereavements – all of these and more might be part of the history of those
working with sick people, and may make them vulnerable.

What is it, in particular, that stresses those working in palliative care?
While this will vary with each individual, there are some common themes
to consider:

- *Feeling helpless*: for example, when symptoms are difficult to
  control, psychological distress doesn't respond to support,
  families are difficult and uncooperative, or the patient has a
  major, uncontrollable haemorrhage.

- *Horror*: some situations in palliative care are horrifying, such as
  visible suppurating cancerous growths, uncontrolled bleeding,
  parts of the face eroded away, patients or families being
  admitted traumatised, or deaths at home where symptoms are
  not controlled. Horror is compounded by feeling helpless but
  made more manageable if action can be taken.

- *Danger*: there may be a perception of danger if a patient or
  relative is aggressive or threatens violence, or if they threaten
  legal action; or if a staff member has a needle stick injury from
  an HIV or hepatitis B positive patient.

- *Overload*: when staff are too busy and tired because of staff sickness, or if a manager carries an excessive workload. Palliative care workers tend to have very high standards and curtailing the care they wish to provide for their dying patients may feel stressful. Making a mistake with the complex drug regimes of dying patients may engender guilt.

- *Reminders*: a particular event reminds the clinician of some distressing incident from their past – bereavement is an obvious example

- *Mortality*: a dead person is a reminder of one's own mortality. While palliative care workers are used to seeing dead people it doesn't mean they are exempt from reflecting on their own ending and fears about how it will be.

- *Staff conflict*: some staff conflict may represent a displacement of distress feelings, including anger, about difficult patients onto other staff. Personal issues such as a complicated divorce, an impending bereavement or financial problems may contribute.

How, then, will stress manifest itself? The possibilities are legion but include:

- *Psychological symptoms*: anxiety, depression, feeling suicidal, tearfulness, panic attacks, insomnia, sleeping all the time, irritability, restlessness, forgetfulness, feeling spaced out, making mistakes, inability to concentrate, indecisiveness.

- *Physical symptoms*: tiredness, palpitations, racing heart, sweating, breathlessness, muscle pains, tingling, headaches, loss of appetite, abdominal pains, diarrhoea, frequent colds, other infections, lump in the throat.

- *Behavioural*: drug and alcohol abuse, family conflict, increased or reduced sexual activity, overeating, anorexia, overspending, personal neglect, isolation, petty theft, errors at work, absenteeism.

It is also possible for a staff member to tip over from feeling stressed into, for example, a major depression. Hence early recognition of the warning signs is needed. And here we come up against a barrier. First, staff do not like to admit that they are stressed, let alone depressed. They see it as a sign of weakness and they feel ashamed to admit their vulnerability. Further, they fear for their job. Doctors are especially caught by this trap. They are trained to be in charge, to know what to do in any crisis, to work long hours without complaint, to be competitive, in other words to be heroic – a superdoc. No wonder they have high levels of stress-related illness. Second, not wanting to be intrusive, their friends and colleagues, or their manager, find it difficult to confront individuals who are showing signs of stress such as heavy drinking. This then is a societal as well as individual issue. If it were a physical illness there would be no problem – there is no stigma attached.

It is only when the entire culture of an organisation changes, when attention to staff stress becomes as important as their salaries, that the barriers mentioned above can be effectively breached. Nevertheless, individuals can still take action for themselves.

SUPPORT MEASURES
Talking informally with friends and colleagues

I remember when I was still training in palliative medicine I went to talk to one of the consultants because I was struggling with my emotional reactions to working with the dying. I remember how she listened quietly and sympathetically without interrupting, and I sensed she understood me. She made a few helpful suggestions without trying to impose anything. I felt better for talking to her. I followed up what we had discussed and this resulted in me altering my approach to working in this field with long-term benefit. I shall always be grateful to her. This sort of interaction is so automatic with most people that they hardly think of it and yet it is a key way that we take care of ourselves. It is the ones who don't do this who are likely to experience problems.

Managerial support

If you have a good manager, consider yourself fortunate. In a way, they have a parental role and we all know how difficult it is to be a good enough parent. Is your manager someone you feel safe enough to go and talk to if you are feeling stressed? Does he have the counselling skills to be supportive? Does he want to be? But, in addition to this, managers are, rightly, expected to intervene if they see you are struggling with your work, showing signs of stress, making mistakes, drinking to excess and so on. This is yet more delicate. How hard it is for managers to talk to their staff about such issues without implying blame and evoking shame. But, it is necessary. It is worse to ignore such symptoms and hope they will go away. It is even worse to deal with them in a cold, critical, dismissive manner, a way that some managers use to protect themselves. And, of course, managers need the support of their own managers. Will they be supported in their attempts to assist a staff member showing signs of stress?

Supervision

Of all the different disciplines, therapy professionals including social workers and counsellors are the best-organised in this area of support. It is part of their culture. It is recognised that this is a skilled intervention needing trained supervisors. Nurses and doctors do not tend to have such a sophisticated system, particularly the latter. And yet this is such a useful way of providing support. When I have facilitated clinical supervision groups with junior doctors, we might start with some difficult clinical issue and yet, after a while, we would be hearing how one of the doctors felt when seeing a patient who was very distressed emotionally, or who was abusive; or perhaps she was wondering how to get through to a withdrawn, depressed patient and feeling frustrated and disempowered. We would explore how she felt and how she might manage the situation using role-play. The meetings would come alive as different ideas were expressed and stories and feelings shared. There would be an intense involvement in the process and a satisfaction in having engaged with not just the intellect, but also the emotional and imaginal dimensions, a deeper and richer experience.

Other clinical meetings

These can provide a degree of support if discussion includes emotional as well as clinical factors. However, they are time-limited and usually have an agenda to be addressed and decisions to be made which restricts the supportive aspect.

Support groups

In 1997 I set up a support group for junior hospice doctors (Feld and Heyse-Moore 2006). I invited a trained counsellor to be the facilitator. Our research showed that the participants found it helpful as a forum for sharing experiences and building relationships. They also appreciated being able to talk about personal or contentious matters in confidence and in having protected time to talk through stressful issues. Sadly, despite its evident value, only 13 per cent of the other hospices we contacted had such groups although 43 per cent informed us they had other informal support measures. Bearing in mind that social workers and, to some extent, nurses have developed this approach more fully, and that there may be few doctors in an individual hospice, a multidisciplinary support group could be a way forward. Nevertheless, they often don't happen which is, perhaps, a reflection on the priorities of individual units and the willingness or otherwise of individuals to participate. After all, while supportive, they may involve looking at uncomfortable personal feelings which some may not wish to do.

Safety

Unlike accident and emergency departments, hospices don't usually have personal safety issues. However, they can occasionally happen and it is only sensible to be prepared. Jackson (2006) suggests various strategies if it seems that aggression is possible:

- *Be prepared*: gather information from the notes, from other staff and, if appropriate, from family members.

- *Look at the setting*: where is the nearest exit? Ensure that the person you are to talk to is not blocking this exit. Are there any potential weapons around? If so, remove them beforehand.

- *Who is going to be present?* a relative or friend may help or worsen the situation. Consider which other members of staff might join you. You might have colleagues waiting outside to come to your assistance if required. If you are visiting a patient or relative at home, consider going in pairs rather than alone. If you think it could be necessary to involve the police, you might consider whether the visit is wise.

- *Be aware of your body language*: to give a message that you are no threat, sit, if it is safe to do so, or stand side-on rather than directly facing the patient. Make eye contact but don't stare, so use a soft, unfocused gaze and look down from time to time. Avoid sudden or large movements of your body such as gestures with your arms. Avoid clenching your fists. If you speak, do so slowly, evenly and softly.

- *Keep quiet and listen*: let him tell his story without interrupting. When he has sounded off and come to a temporary halt, then reflect back something of what he said and invite him to tell you more if he so wishes. While it may not be possible to concur with his wish to be violent, it is still possible to empathise with how upsetting the situation was that brought on the angry feelings. Often, this process by itself will be enough to restore calmness. You have heard him out and respected his viewpoint and it may then be possible to look at constructive solutions to his issue.

- *Keep observing the other person's body language*: look out for signs of impending violence, such as erratic movements, if she restlessly paces about, or if her voice becomes louder and more aggressive.

- If it is clear that violence is a possibility try to stay as self-aware as you can as this will help you not to be overtaken by panic. Focus on your breathing, your chest rising and falling; consciously feel the ground under your feet. These are ways of staying grounded.

- While encouraging the patient or relative to tell his story and keeping your body language non-confrontational, look around for an exit strategy. Avoid having your legs crossed as this could slow your escape.

- If all else fails and violence is impending, RUN! There is no shame in this; misplaced heroics will only get you into trouble.

- These can be traumatic encounters, so afterwards debrief with a colleague and, if necessary, a counsellor.

- Ensure accurate, factual notes are kept for legal purposes.

Counselling

Why might a palliative care worker see a counsellor? This could either be short-term for self-limiting issues such as stress at work or a recent bereavement, or it could be longer term if work-related stress has been a trigger uncovering deeper psychological issues such as childhood traumas. However, here again we encounter the barrier already mentioned. Counselling may be seen as implying mental health problems which are vigorously rejected – 'I'm not crazy; I don't need to see a trick cyclist.'[1] There is a fear of being identified with the insane. Fortunately, this view is changing, albeit gradually. In the end, it is an individual's choice; there is no value in going for counselling under duress. For it to be helpful, it must be a cooperative venture.

Some hospices make counselling available to their staff – for example, six sessions free of charge. Many general practice surgeries provide time-limited counselling. NHS psychiatric services are grossly overstretched with long waiting lists and so not a realistic option. MIND, the mental health charity, provides free professional counselling through their local branches (see the Resources section at the end of this book for details). The final possibility is private counselling, the cost of which can be an issue for those on low incomes. Some counsellors use a sliding scale based on the client's income for the fees they charge. Assuming you wish to go for counselling, how do you choose the right counsellor? It is worth doing some research beforehand. The internet is a ready source of information on the various types of counselling available. See which one appeals to you. Some practitioners are integrative which means they combine more than one school of therapy synergistically in their practice. To find a practitioner, possibilities include word of mouth or again the internet. The British Association for Counselling and Psychotherapy (BACP), for example, lists all its members including their psychological approach to therapy. When you meet a counsellor for the first time, you need to ensure that you can get on together, that you can work with her. There is no point in starting counselling with someone you don't like. Furthermore, you may have questions you would like to ask her, about how she works, for example. The first meeting is really a mutual assessment from which either side may withdraw, or to agree a contract of the number of sessions and what the aims of the counselling work together are to be.

There are no set rules as to how counselling progresses. It depends on the individual. You may feel better quickly simply by being listened to well. You may experience more emotions than usual. You may come up against a block and feel numb instead. Your counsellor is there to help you

1   Slang for psychiatrist.

negotiate these various processes. Most people appreciate the support, the holding, that working with a counsellor provides. And it can be very hard work. It can also be engrossing and enjoyable. Furthermore, it leads almost inevitably to a deeper awareness and understanding of your self. It is tempting to look for a quick fix. It may be more helpful to see it as part of your life journey where the counsellor acts as a guide and support when you get stuck or overwhelmed, much as an explorer might need a guide when traversing uncharted territory.

Treatment and time off

If you have decided, after discussion with your general practitioner to take psychotropic drugs, say for depression, then consider combining this approach with counselling. Recovery from depression is quicker when both modalities are used together. Drugs will relieve the symptoms but they can't address ongoing issues such as work problems or an impending divorce.

If you need time off, consider how to use it. Regular exercise is a known antidote to depression. Stress-related conditions may be exhausting, so getting enough sleep to allow your body to recover is important. Depression and grief may lead to a loss of appetite and loss of weight; hence you need to ensure you eat enough, even if it is a struggle. Having something to occupy your mind is helpful and counteracts excessive introspection. Norman Cousins (1979), in his book *Anatomy of an Illness* about his recovery from severe ankylosing spondylitis, described using humour, in the shape of Marx Brothers films, reruns of *Candid Camera*, and humorous books. He found his pain would be alleviated and, even more remarkable, his blood tests (the erythrocyte sedimentation rate) improved. When you do feel better, it may be taxing to change from being quietly at home to returning full-time to work, so a gradual return may be appropriate especially if you have been away a long time. If your manager wants you to be seen by the occupational health department, remember they are not out to fire you; rather, it's the opposite. They will look for every way they can to get you back to work, but also to ensure you don't return before you're ready. Furthermore, if for some reason you cannot return to your previous responsibilities, they will recommend an alternative that suits your present capabilities.

The job

If there is some aspect of your job that you find stressful, talk with your manager about ways of changing this. If the job really isn't suiting you, it may be beneficial to consider looking for a different post that fits your needs better.

Meditation

I have already written about this in the clinical context (see Chapter 5) detailing various types of meditation practice. When LeShan (1999) asked a group of scientists why they meditated, one man came up with an answer which all agreed with: it is like coming home. If you are under pressure, with its consequent outpouring of the stress hormones adrenaline and cortisol, then the physiological relaxation response of meditation will act as a welcome counter to this hyperaroused state.

I remember doing a relaxation meditation with a group of hospice staff. Before that, they were, by their own admission, in high gear physiologically, prepared to meet the demands of a busy day. As we went through the meditation, I could feel the tension in the room slowly melt away. By the end, they had slowed right down, felt calm, relaxed and were struck by the difference before and after. Their experience taught them that this could be a useful antidote to the strains of working with the dying.

If you think this is for you, then here are some suggestions:

- It is important that you choose a type of meditation practice that suits you. If you're not sure, it's worth trying one method for at least a fortnight to get a sense of its suitability for you.

- The usual advice is to meditate for about 20–30 minutes once or twice a day at particular times that you have decided such as morning and evening. It may be necessary for those not used to meditation to start with a shorter time and build up gradually.

- Sitting upright is recommended as it aids concentration.

- The eyes can be shut or kept half closed and looking softly at a point a few feet in front of you.

- Rest your hands lightly on your lap.

- You can sit in a chair or on a cushion on the ground cross-legged. The lotus position is fine for those with flexible joints but not for the rest of us who are more tightly knit.

Meditation can be hard work. It requires persistence to sit quietly and stay with awareness of your breathing. Your mind will inevitably wander – the many thoughts that arise unbidden to our consciousness have been compared to unruly wild horses – and part of the practice is to bring back your attention gently and repeatedly to your chosen focus. Nevertheless, even meditations that feel boring, distracted and restless will still have a beneficial effect in your everyday life.

Playing

When Carl Jung was going through a crisis in his life, he decided to spend time sitting on the shores of the lake where he had built a house, playing, as a child would, with mud, sticks and stones, and building a model village. Engrossed in this game, he felt instinctively that this would be therapeutic for him, as indeed it was (Jung 1983, pp.197–9). All of us play – it makes no difference that we are adult. We play at sports, play card games, play with our children, play a musical instrument and go to the theatre to see a play, for example. It is something we do for sheer pleasure and, not surprisingly, it is restorative, healing and renewing. I can recall a pathologist who used to do post mortems for a hospice, who, in striking contrast, collected Chinese porcelain. Different hospice workers I have come across have belonged to choirs, played squash, travelled widely, been keen amateur cooks, bird-watchers, walkers, gardeners, musicians, writers or poets. As the adage goes, all work and no play has a seriously detrimental effect on Jack's health. So what is your way of playing, what gives you pleasure? The possibilities are many. However, it does require a degree of determination. To say that you would like to take up such and such but you just haven't got the time, is not enough. This is the dragging voice of your inner critic calling you back to the treadmill. Instead, make time, factor it in. You have to be serious about enjoying yourself. After all, it is for your health and you are worth it.

Conclusion

In setting out approaches to using counselling skills in palliative care and discussing their use in various areas of care of the dying such as breaking bad news or emotional support, I have tried to show that they have an essential place which is different from, but complementary to, the Western medical model – the Asklepian and Hippocratic schools working in synchrony. I have also discussed the toll that this work can take on its practitioners and hence the importance of good staff support.

We will all eventually follow the same path as the many patients described in this book. In that sense, they are our teachers. They have experienced something we have yet to encounter. For all our academic learning about dying, we know less than they did about what it is actually like to die.

Sometimes, using counselling skills when working with the dying is difficult and frustrating. Patients may be confused, forgetful, and not able to concentrate for long. There isn't enough time to address long-term psychological issues. Their condition may change rapidly. They may die at any time. Sometimes, though, it flies:

> We become explorers immersed in the grandest and most complex of pursuits – the development and maintenance of the human mind. Hand in hand with patients, we savour the pleasure of great discoveries – the 'aha' experience when disparate ideational fragments suddenly slide smoothly together into coherence. At other times we are midwife to the birth of something new, liberating and elevating. We watch our patients let go of old self-defeating patterns, detach from ancient grievances, develop zest for living, learn to love us, and, through that act, turn lovingly to others. It is a joy to see others open the taps to their own founts of wisdom. Sometimes I feel like a guide escorting patients

through the rooms of their own house. What a treat it is to watch them open doors to rooms never before entered, discover new wings of their house containing parts in exile – wise, beautiful and creative pieces of identity. (Yalom 2001, p.258)

References

Achteberg, J. (2002) *Imagery in Healing*. Boston MA and London: Shambhala.

American Psychiatric Association (2000) *Diagnostic and Statistical Manual of Mental Disorders*. Fourth revision, text revision. Washington DC: American Psychiatric Association.

Assagioli, R. (1975) *Psychosynthesis*. Wellingborough: Turnstone Press.

Assagioli, R. (1984) *The Act of Will*. Wellingborough: Turnstone Press.

Axline, V. (1971) *Dibs In Search of Self*. Harmondsworth: Pelican.

Barasch, M.I. (1993) *The Healing Path*. New York: Penguin Arkana.

Bauby, J-D. (1998) *The Diving Bell and the Butterfly*. London: Fourth Estate.

Bayliss, J. (2004) *Counselling Skills in Palliative Care*. Salisbury: Quay Books.

Beck, A.T. (1989) *Cognitive Therapy and the Emotional Disorders*. London: Penguin.

Benson, H. (1996) *Timeless Healing*. London: Simon & Schuster.

Bluebond-Langner, M. (1978) *The Private Worlds of Dying Children*. Princeton, NJ: Princeton University Press.

BMA News (2007) 'One of life's hardest lessons.' 30 June, p.19.

Bradshaw, J. (1988) *Healing the Shame that Binds You*. Deerfield Beach, FL: Health Communication Inc.

Breitbart, W., Chochinov, H.M. and Passik S.D. (2004) 'Psychiatric Symptoms in Palliative Medicine.' In D. Doyle, G. Hanks, N. Cherny and K. Calman (eds) *Oxford Textbook of Palliative Medicine*. 3rd edition. Oxford: Oxford University Press.

Buber, M. (1958) *I and Thou*. Edinburgh: T&T Clark.

Campbell, J. (1990) *The Hero's Journey*. Novato, CA: New World Library.

Cardinal, M. (1993) *The Words to Say It*. London: Women's Press.

Carnegie, D. (1988) *How to Win Friends and Influence People*. London: Cedar.

Carter, R. (1999) *Mapping the Mind*. London: Seven Dials.

Chatwin, B. (1987) *The Songlines*. London: Picador.

Chödrön, P. (1997) *When Things Fall Apart*. London: Element.

Cousins, N. (1979) *Anatomy of an Illness*. New York: Bantam Books.

Cornish, P. (1994) 'In memory of Harriet.' *View 1*, 16–19.

Culley, S. and Bond, T. (2004) *Integrative Counselling Skills in Action*. 2nd edition. London: Sage.

d'Ardenne, P. and Mahtani, A. (1989) *Transcultural Counselling in Action*. London: Sage.

Darwin, C. (1872) *The Expression of Emotions in Animals and Man*. London: Murray.

Dass, R. and Gorman, P. (1986) *How Can I Help*. London: Rider.

de Hennezel, M. (1997) *Intimate Death*. London: Warner Books.

Endicott, J. (1984) 'Measurement of depression in patients with cancer.' *Cancer 53*, 10 (suppl), 2243–9.

Feld, J. and Heyse-Moore, L. (2006) 'An evaluation of a support group for junior doctors working in palliative care.' *American Journal of Hospice and Palliative Medicine 23*, 4, 287–96.

Ferrucci, P. (1982) *What We May Be*. Wellingborough: Turnstone Press.

Fisher, R., Ury, W. and Patton, B. (1992) *Getting to Yes*. 2nd edition. London: Random House.

Frankl, V.E. (2004) *Man's Search for Meaning*. London: Rider (original work published 1946).

Freshwater, D. and Robertson, C. (2002) *Emotions and Needs*. Buckingham: Open University Press.

General Medical Council (2006) *Good Medical Practice*. London: General Medical Council.

Goldie, L. and Desmarais, J. (2005) *Psychotherapy and the Treatment of Cancer*. London: Routledge.

Graves, R. (1992) *The Greek Myths*. (Complete edition.) London: Penguin.

Harvey, A. and Matousek, M. (1994) *Dialogues With a Modern Mystic*. Wheaton, IL: Quest.

Herbert, M. (1996) *Supporting Bereaved and Dying Children and Their Parents*. Leicester: BPS Books.

Hesse, H. (1991) *Siddhartha*. London: Picador.

Heyse-Moore, L. (1996) 'On spiritual pain in the dying.' *Mortality 1*, 3, 297–315.

Heyse-Moore, L. (2007) 'Dying to talk.' *Therapy Today 18*, 5, 11–14.

Heyse-Moore, L. and Johnson-Bell, V. (1987) 'Can doctors accurately predict the life expectancy of patients with terminal cancer?' *Palliative Medicine 1*, 2, 165–6.

Hillman, J. (1992) *Revisioning Psychology*. New York: HarperPerennial.

House of Lords (1994) *Select Committee on Medical Ethics Report*. House of Lords paper 21-I. London: HMSO.

Jackson, C. (2006) *Shut Up and Listen – a Brief Guide to Clinical Communication Skills*. Dundee: University of Dundee.

Jacobs, M. (1998) *The Presenting Past*. 2nd edition. Maidenhead: Open University Press.

Jacoby, M. (1984) *The Analytic Encounter*. Toronto: Inner City.

Johnson, R.A. (1986) *Inner Work*. New York: HarperSanFrancisco.

Jones, A. (ed.) (1966) *The Jerusalem Bible: New Testament*. London: Darton, Longman & Todd.

Jung, C.G. (ed.) (1964) *Man and his Symbols*. London: Aldus.

Jung, C.G. (1969) 'Psychology and Religion: West and East.' In H. Read, M. Fordham and G. Adler (eds) (1953–1979) *The Collected Works of C.G. Jung Vol. 11*. London: Routledge.

Jung, C.G. (1983) *Memories, Dreams and Reflections*. London: Flamingo.

Kabat-Zinn, J. (1990) *Full Catastrophe Living*. New York: Delta Publishing.

Kearney, M. (1996) *Mortally Wounded*. Dublin: Marino.

Keen, S. (1974) 'The golden mean of Roberto Assagioli.' *Psychology Today 10*, 6, 96–104.

Kipling, R. (1902) 'I Keep Six Honest Serving Men.' In P. Keating (ed.) (1999) *Rudyard Kipling: Selected Poems*. London: Penguin.

Kübler-Ross, E. (1969) *On Death and Dying*. London: Routledge.

Lawrence, D.H. (1994) 'Healing.' In *D.H. Lawrence: The Complete Poems*. Ware: Wordsworth.

LeShan, L. (1994) *Cancer as a Turning Point*. Revised edition. London: Plume.

LeShan, L. (1999) *How to Meditate*. Boston, MA: Backbay Books.

Levine, P.A. (1997) *Waking the Tiger*. Berkeley, CA: North Atlantic Books.

Mindell, A. (1994) *Coma: the Dreambody Near Death*. London: Arkana.

Moore, T. (1994) *Care of the Soul*. New York: HarperPerennial.

Moorey, S. and Greer, S. (2002) *Cognitive Behavioural Therapy for Patients with Cancer*. Oxford: Oxford University Press.

Mukherjee, E. and Foster, R. (2008) 'The Mental Capacity Act 2007 and capacity assessments: a guide for the non-psychiatrist.' *Clinical Medicine 8*, 1, 65–9.

National Collaborating Centre for Mental Health (NCCMH) (2004) *Depression: Management of Depression in Primary and Secondary Care.* Leicester: British Psychological Society, and London: Gaskell.

Pullman, P. (1995) *Northern Lights.* London: Scholastic Press.

Puri, B.K., Laking, P.J. and Treasaden, I.H. (1996) *Textbook of Psychiatry.* London: Churchill Livingstone.

Reber, A.S. and Reber, E.S. (2001) *Dictionary of Psychology.* 3rd edition. London: Penguin.

Remen, R.N. (1997) *Kitchen Table Wisdom.* London: Pan.

Robertson, C. (1997) *An Integrative Framework.* Unpublished.

Rogers, C. (1961) *On Becoming a Person.* London: Constable.

Rycroft, C. (1995) *Critical Dictionary of Psychoanalysis.* 2nd edition. London: Penguin.

Satir, V. (1972) *Peoplemaking.* Palo Alto, CA: Science and Behaviour Books.

Shakespeare, W. (1905) *Macbeth.* In W.J. Craig (ed.) *Shakespeare: Complete Works.* London: Oxford University Press.

Shapiro, F. and Forrest, M.S. (2004) *EMDR.* New York: Basic Books.

St John of the Cross (1976) *Dark Night of the Soul.* Tunbridge Wells: Burns & Oates.

Storr, A. (ed.) (1998) *The Essential Jung.* London: Fontana Press.

Tolkien, J.R.R. (1966) *The Hobbit.* London: George Allen & Unwin. (Original work published 1937).

Vachon, M.L.S. (1995) 'Staff stress in hospital/palliative care: a review.' *Palliative Medicine 9,* 91–122.

Varley, S. (1985) *Badger's Parting Gifts.* London: Fontana Picture Lions.

Vining, R.M. (1995) 'Assessing risk of suicide.' *British Medical Journal 310,* 126–7.

Winnicott, D.W. (1988) *Babies and Their Mothers.* London: Free Association Books.

Worden, J.W. (2003) *Grief Counselling and Grief Therapy.* 3rd edition. London: Routledge.

Yalom, I. (2001) *The Gift of Therapy.* London: Piatkus.

Recommended Reading List

PALLIATIVE CARE COUNSELLING

Bayliss, J. (2004) *Counselling Skills in Palliative Care.* Salisbury: Quay Books.

de Hennezel, M. (1997) *Intimate Death.* London: Warner Books.

Goldie, L. and Desmarais, J. (2005) *Psychotherapy and the Treatment of Cancer.* London: Routledge.

Kearney, M. (1996) *Mortally Wounded.* Dublin: Marino.

Kübler-Ross, E. (1969) *On Death and Dying.* New York: Macmillan.

LeShan, L. (1994) *Cancer as a Turning Point.* Revised edition. London: Plume.

Levine, S. (1986) *Who Dies?* Dublin: Gateway.

Remen, R.N. (1997) *Kitchen Table Wisdom.* London: Pan.

GENERAL COUNSELLING AND PSYCHOTHERAPY

Culley, S. and Bond, T. (2004) *Integrative Counselling Skills in Action.* 2nd edition. London: Sage.

Frankl, V.E. (2004) *Man's Search for Meaning.* London: Rider.

Gerhardt, S. (2004) *Why Love Matters.* Hove: Brunner-Routledge.

Jung, C.G. (ed.) (1964) *Man and his Symbols.* London: Aldus.

Levine, P.A. (1997) *Waking the Tiger.* Berkeley, CA: North Atlantic Books.

Miller, A. (1997) *The Drama of Being a Child.* Revised edition. London: Virago.

Rogers, C. (1961) *On Becoming a Person.* London: Constable.

Satir, V. (1972) *Peoplemaking.* Palo Alto, CA: Science and Behaviour Books.

Yalom, I. (2001) *The Gift of Therapy.* London: Piatkus.

MEDITATION AND VISUALISATION

Ferrucci, P. (1982) *What We May Be.* Wellingborough: Turnstone Press.

Johnson, R.A. (1986) *Inner Work.* New York: HarperSanFrancisco.

LeShan, L. (1999) *How to Meditate.* Boston, MA: Back Bay Books.

Kabat-Zinn, J. (1990) *Full Catastrophe Living.* New York: Delta Publishing.

PERSONAL ACCOUNTS

Albom, M. (2003) *Tuesdays with Morrie.* London: Time Warner Books.

Axline, V. (1971) *Dibs In Search of Self.* Harmondsworth: Pelican.

Bauby, J-D. (1998) *The Diving Bell and the Butterfly.* London: Fourth Estate.

Cardinal, M. (1993) *The Words to Say It.* London: The Women's Press.

Cousins, N. (1979) *Anatomy of an Illness.* New York: Bantam Books.

Jung, C. (1983) *Memories, Dreams and Reflections*. London: Flamingo.

Schreiber, F.R. (1974) *Sybil*. London: Penguin.

BOOKS FOR YOUNGER CHILDREN

Burningham, J. (2003) *Granpa*. London: Red Fox.

Clark, E.C. (2006) *Up in Heaven*. London: Andersen Press.

Sanders, B. (2006) *Talking about Death and Dying*. London: Aladdin Books.

Varley, S. (1985) *Badger's Parting Gifts*. London: Fontana Picture Lions.

BOOKS FOR OLDER CHILDREN AND TEENAGERS

Bowler, T. (2006) *River Boy*. Oxford: Oxford University Press.

Lewis, C.S. (1964) *The Chronicles of Narnia*. (7 volumes) Harmondsworth: Puffin.

Pullman, P. (2001) *His Dark Materials Trilogy*. London: Scholastic Press.

Resources

(All websites accessed 25 June 2008)

ACT Association for Children's Palliative Care
Orchard House, Orchard Lane
Bristol BS1 5DT
0117 922 1556
www.act.org.uk
Children's palliative care promotion, support and information.

British Association for Counselling and Psychotherapy
BACP House, 15 St John's Business Park
Lutterworth, Leicestershire LE17 4HB
0870 443 5252
www.bacp.co.uk
Professional association and regulatory body. Information on counselling centres and individual therapists' register. Research and education journals.

Buddhist Hospice Trust
31 Weir Gardens
Rayleigh, Essex SS6 7TQ
01268 775521
www.buddhisthospice.org.uk
Palliative care support from a Buddhist perspective.

Cancer Black Care
79 Acton Lane
London NW10 8UT
020 8961 4151
www.cancerblackcare.org
Cancer support service for the black and ethnic minority community.

Cancer Counselling Trust
1 Noel Road
London N1 8HQ
020 7704 1137
www.cctrust.org.uk
Free professional counselling support for anyone experiencing the distress of cancer – e.g. patients, family, professionals.

CHAI Cancer Care Hendon Centre
144–146 Great North Way
London NW4 1EH
020 8202 2211
www.chaicancercare.org
Cancer support services for the Jewish community.

Cruse Bereavement Care
Cruse House, 126 Sheen Road
Richmond, Surrey TW9 1UR
020 8939 9530
www.crusebereavementcare.org.uk
Bereavement support and training.

Help the Hospices
Hospice House, 34–44 Britannia Street
London WC1X 9JG
020 7520 8200
www.helpthehospices.org.uk
National hospice charity – training, education, information, fund-raising.

Hospice Information
St Christopher's Hospice
51–59 Lawrie Park Road
London SE26 6DZ
0870 903 3903
www.hospiceinformation.info
Information service on all aspects of palliative care, including bookshop.

Karnac Bookshop
118 Finchley Road
London NW3 5HT
020 7431 1075
www.karnacbooks.com
Bookseller specialising in psychological therapies.

Macmillan Cancer Support
89 Albert Embankment
London SE1 7UQ
020 7840 7840 (7841 for their CancerLine)
www.macmillan.org.uk
Funds palliative care posts and buildings. Grants to patients in need financially. (Now incorporates Cancerbackup.)

Motor Neurone Disease Association
PO Box 246
Northampton NN1 2PR
01604 250505
www.mndassociation.org
Support organisation for patients with motor neurone disease.

MIND
15-19 Broadway
London E15 4BQ
0845 766 0163 (infoline)
www.mind.org.uk
Mental health charity. Information. Support. Counselling.

Penny Brohn Cancer Care (formerly the Bristol Cancer Help Centre)
Chapel Pill Lane
Pill, Bristol BS20 0HH
www.pennybrohncancercare.org
Complementary approach to cancer support working in cooperation with orthodox medical treatment.
Education resource centre.

Re.Vision
Centre for Integrative Psychosynthesis Counselling and Psychotherapy
97 Brondesbury Road
London NW6 6RY
020 8357 8881
www.re-vision.org.uk
Therapy training centre and counselling service.

The Terrence Higgins Trust
314–320 Gray's Inn Road
London WC1X 8DP
020 7812 1600
www.tht.org.uk
Support, information and guidance on HIV infection, AIDS and sexual health. 'Buddy' support
system.

United Kingdom Council for Psychotherapy
2nd floor, Edward House, 2 Wakling Street
London EC1V 7LT
020 7014 9955
www.psychotherapy.org.uk
Regulatory body promoting practice, research, education and training in psychotherapy.

Subject Index

Author Index

Lightning Source UK Ltd.
Milton Keynes UK
24 May 2010

154627UK00002B/13/P